Guiding Doctors in Managing their Careers

A TOOLKIT FOR TUTORS, TRAINERS, MENTORS AND APPRAISERS

Ruth Chambers
Director of GP Postgraduate Education
West Midlands Deanery

Kay Mohanna
General Practitioner
Principal Lecturer in Medical Education
Staffordshire University

Andrew Thornett
General Practitioner
Senior Clinical Lecturer
Staffordshire University

Steve Field
Regional Postgraduate Medical Dean
West Midlands Deanery
Chair of the Education Network
Royal College of General Practitioners

Radcliffe Publishing
Oxford • Seattle

Radcliffe Publishing Ltd
18 Marcham Road
Abingdon
Oxon OX14 1AA
United Kingdom

www.radcliffe-oxford.com
Electronic catalogue and worldwide online ordering facility.

British Library Cataloguing in Publication Data

A catalogue record for this book is available from the British Library.

ISBN 10 1 85775 611 8
ISBN 13 978 1 85775 611 1

Typeset by Advance Typesetting Ltd, Oxford
Printed and bound by TJ International Ltd, Padstow, Cornwall

Contents

Preface

This toolkit will help all those whose job or role puts them in the position of providing careers information, advice or guidance to medical students or doctors at some stage in their career. You might be a general practitioner (GP) or clinical tutor, a GP trainer or an appraiser. You might advise doctors in their foundation years or in other training programmes, or doctors whose performance is giving concern. You might work for a university, a deanery, a trust or other organisation, within or outside the NHS. If you hold any of these roles, or expect to do so, then this toolkit is for you. It will help you know what is expected of you, give you an opportunity to reflect on your current knowledge and skills, and enable you to develop effective information- and advice-giving skills.

Medical students or doctors may need careers information or advice as their career evolves, or at specific points in their career where choices have to be made. Any such information or advice should be part of a co-ordinated system which is linked into the education programme or continuing professional development underpinning their training or professional lives. It should take account of NHS service needs, but in an open and transparent way, so that anyone receiving careers advice can understand and appreciate the context.

The *Modernising Medical Careers* initiative has highlighted the traditional paucity of careers support for medical students and doctors in training and, by generalising, for established doctors too. Simply teaching students and doctors how to undertake career planning and manage their own career will go a long way to enabling them to make the right career choices for their personality and circumstances. Challenging them to review their situation, formulate aspirations and plan their career track is key to their career and job satisfaction. Putting them back in touch with the values and beliefs that brought them into medicine, and providing opportunities to diversify and develop, should help to retain doctors in practice. Doing all this as part of a local strategy that is co-ordinated by the deanery is central to the vision for a career management model for the future.[1] This toolkit will help you to play your part in achieving this vision. It will help you to appreciate what is expected of you and prepare, whatever your role or responsibility, for medical students' or doctors' development.

Ruth Chambers
Kay Mohanna
Andrew Thornett
Steve Field
December 2005

Reference

1 Modernising Medical Careers Working Groups for Career Management (2005) *Career Management: an approach for medical schools, deaneries, royal colleges and trusts*. The Stationery Office, London.

About the authors

Ruth Chambers has been a GP for more than 20 years. Her previous experience has encompassed a wide range of research and educational activities and she has been involved in promoting career development for many years. She is currently Director of GP Postgraduate Education at the West Midlands Deanery and Professor of Primary Care at Staffordshire University. Ruth has researched and written about the need for medical careers support services and run career guidance skills training around the UK. She ran a support scheme for doctors and dentists in Staffordshire for nearly ten years, with career counselling as a component resource. One of her most formative experiences was an in-depth career review that led to her diversifying within an academic/clinical career.

Kay Mohanna has made several changes in her life and career without the benefit of objective careers advice or guidance. She undertook research as the Royal College of General Practitioners' Midland Faculty young practitioners' fellow in 1997–98 to reveal the need for career support for GPs in the early years of practice, and produced a resource booklet. During her academic career as a principal lecturer in Medical Education at Staffordshire University, Kay has met and helped many doctors with their career development. Their experiences illustrate their need for interested careers advisers with objective and up-to-date information about alternative career pathways. Kay has co-authored a book with Ruth about medical career guidance, and run national seminars for doctors aiding their career decisions.

Andrew Thornett is a GP in Tamworth, with postgraduate training and qualifications in psychiatry and child health. He trained as a GP in Nottinghamshire, before working in Southampton as a clinical research fellow. He then spent a year in rural and remote South Australia before joining Staffordshire University as Senior Lecturer in Medical Education. Andrew has a particular interest in the quality of careers advice that doctors have available to make informed choices that suit their personal and social commitments, as well as meeting their professional goals. His current research interests include exploring the competencies that GP careers advisers should demonstrate.

Steve Field is Regional Postgraduate Medical Dean at the West Midlands Deanery, Honorary Professor of Medical Education at the University of Warwick, Honorary Professor at the University of Birmingham and Chair of the Education Network, Royal College of General Practitioners. He has been a GP since 1986 and continues to work part-time as a GP in inner-city Birmingham. He has been vice-chair of the Committee of GP Education Directors (COGPED), chair of the Implementation Committee for the UK GP Registrar Scheme and chair of the National Summative Assessment Board for General Practice. Steve is a founder member of the Postgraduate Medical Education and Training Board and chairs the Department of Health's Modernising Medical Careers Delivery Board. Despite all of that, he continues to be actively involved in teaching and learning, with a particular interest in communication skills and assessment methods.

Judi Thorley is a senior nurse and modern matron at a community hospital in North Staffordshire. She joined Ruth and Andy as a researcher for a short-term research and development post to study GPs' perspectives of careers support.

Dedication

This book is offered in homage to the extensive contribution Dr Rhona MacDonald has made to promoting opportunities for doctors' career development and fulfilment, in her several years as editor of Career Focus for the *British Medical Journal*. Under Rhona's leadership with support from Jackie Connor the Director and other colleagues such as Peter Cross and Dr Graham Easton, Career Focus has become a key national source of careers information, improving the career lot of many doctors. Rhona's special interest in enabling doctors experiencing disadvantage to progress their careers has led to many articles and information guides that have truly supported equality and valued diversity, and made an impact on the medical establishment.

Glossary of terms

Career consultation: 'targeted activities designed to respond to the particular needs and concerns of the individual, with an ability and confirmed level of demonstrable competence to manage and support career crises.'[1]

Career counselling: is an umbrella term for the process of enabling somebody to evaluate their current situation and identify what steps are needed in order to change. It will usually include identification of a person's strengths and weaknesses in relation to work options and may also include careers information.[2]

Career exploration: 'activities designed to provide accurate, accessible information, specialty workforce profiling and reflective career thinking space for medical students, doctors in training and more experienced clinicians.'[1]

Career facilitation: 'activities designed to provide programmed personal interventions and initiatives and appropriate facilitated peer group networks in the medical school and into the training years which align personal awareness of career options, aptitude, strengths and career interests with that required of doctors.'[1]

Careers guidance: is personal and directive, and provides *advice* within the context of the opportunities that are available.[2]

Careers information: covers the facts about the qualifications and experience needed for alternative career pathways and the opportunities that there are for career progression. That is, the number and type of posts available at a particular level and in a particular specialty and details of the qualifications and training necessary.[2]

Career management: this covers the whole process of how an individual doctor progresses towards set goals and aims, career exploration activities, career facilitation and career consultation. The term is used in relation to individual doctor or organisational perspectives. This includes curriculum initiatives, career resources, medical workforce and labour market intelligence, learning experiences, employer perspectives and personal development activities.[1]

Coaching: is the process of motivating, encouraging and helping an individual to improve their skills, knowledge and attitudes in a framework of goal setting and achievement.[3]

Mentoring: is the process whereby an experienced, highly regarded empathic person (the mentor) guides another individual (the mentee) in the development and re-examination of their own ideas, learning and personal and professional development.[4,5]

Reflection: is the process whereby people actively deliberate on their performance or the care they deliver and identify their strengths and weaknesses (as individuals or in groups).

Skills escalator: is an approach to developing careers in the NHS through a supportive culture and infrastructure. The vision of a modernised NHS is for staff to have a range of options for developing and extending their careers, supported by learning and development opportunities. Getting people on the escalator means attracting a wide range of people to work within the NHS by offering advice and help within a variety of career and training stages. Enabling staff to move on the escalator is about encouraging staff to renew and extend their skills and knowledge to gain stimulating careers through a strategy of lifelong learning.[6]

References

1 Modernising Medical Careers Working Groups for Career Management (2005) *Career Management: an approach for medical schools, deaneries, royal colleges and trusts*. The Stationery Office, London.

2 Chambers R, Mohanna K and Field S (2000) *Opportunities and Options in Medical Careers*. Radcliffe Medical Press, Oxford.

3 Binding C and Sowden D (2004) *Making Sense of the Medical Career Maze – a UK consultation document and proposal for implementation in Trent*. Trent Postgraduate Deanery, University of Nottingham, Nottingham.

4 Chambers R, Mohanna K, Wakley G and Wall D (2004) *Demonstrating Your Competence 1. Healthcare teaching*. Radcliffe Medical Press, Oxford.

5 Standing Committee on Postgraduate Medical and Dental Education (1998) *An Enquiry into Mentoring; supporting doctors and dentists at work*. Standing Committee on Postgraduate Medical and Dental Education, London.

6 Department of Health (2004) *Skills Escalator. Achieving your potential*. Department of Health, London.

1

Effective careers information, guidance and career counselling – for doctors and medical students

Ruth Chambers

There are over 65 medical specialties with varying training requirements and programmes. Then there are subspecialties, extended roles such as in teaching or management, academic and research posts, differing healthcare settings such as urban or rural practice and type of hospital or general practice.[1,2] With all this complexity, many medical students or doctors need help in actively selecting and managing their careers. They may require information about the variety of careers available and how to access them. Or they may require more individualised help, identifying the factors that are important to them in selecting a discipline or new specialist area and picturing their priorities in terms of skills, interests and what motivates them. Doctors in established careers may want to reassess their career to date or explore new opportunities, or address gaps in their knowledge or skills or experience.

Thinking of the medical workforce

The structure of the medical workforce has changed dramatically since the early 1990s. The number of consultants, including directors of public health, has increased by an average 5% per year from 17 600 in 1993 to 30 400 in 2004, in England.[3] General practitioner (GP) numbers have increased too, but by a much smaller percentage, an average 1.4% per year from 28 500 in 1993 to 34 000 in 2004.[4] When these figures are calculated as whole-time equivalents, the increase is much the same for consultants, but an average increase of only 0.8% for GPs since 1993. The proportion of female consultants grew from 18% in 1994 to 28% in 2004.[3]

We have many more doctors coming to work in the UK who have trained overseas these days. Overseas trained doctors make up a third of UK Senior House Officer (SHO) posts. It is not yet clear how many doctors from the new European Union (EU) countries will apply for jobs in the UK. The General Medical Council (GMC) offers 10 000 places for taking the second stage of the Professional and Linguistic Assessment Board (PLAB) exam for doctors from outside the EU, every year. No mechanism is in place to regulate the numbers of doctors taking PLAB to match likely training vacancies. So there is a surplus of doctors who have passed PLAB 2, have limited registration from the GMC and a work permit, who are seeking their first post in a training grade. About three-quarters find a job within six months of passing their PLAB tests.[5] Some are refugee doctors. The British Medical Association (BMA) refugee doctor database has more than a thousand refugee doctors registered on it.

There are several options for international medical recruitment. The NHS international fellowship programme offers two year placements in the NHS and is particularly aimed at experienced senior doctors in certain specialties that are in high demand.[6] International doctors' induction courses help non-UK medical graduates with little or no knowledge of the UK or the NHS. They are held in most deaneries as 2–4-day courses.

Modernising Medical Careers expects careers information, advice and guidance to be readily available

The *Modernising Medical Careers* (MMC) initiative has significantly changed the nature and content of medical training.[7] Chapter 2 describes the MMC initiative in detail. Appropriate careers information, advice and guidance for all doctors in the foundation years are integral to the MMC reforms. Many of the arrangements for supporting career management for doctors in training (and medical students) can be generalised to doctors established in career specialties too to help sustain their long-term interest in a medical career.

Lack of careers information, advice and guidance

Most established doctors report that they have never received any careers guidance or counselling, and any advice that they have received has been mainly informal and *ad hoc*. The inadequacy of the extent and scope of careers information, advice, guidance and counselling available to medical students, doctors in training and throughout their careers has been widely publicised by academics and professional bodies.[1,8–12] Over half of the doctors in training and final year medical students responding to one survey undertaken by the National Institute for Careers Education and Counselling (NICEC) reported that they were quite or very dissatisfied with the career advice and guidance they had received, whilst only one-sixth were quite or very satisfied. Most of these respondents agreed that what they knew about careers in medicine came from personal experience.[8] A local study in the West Midlands had similar findings of a scarcity of careers support services being available to GPs and other primary care staff.[13]

Findings from the BMA cohort study of doctors qualifying in 1995 emphasised the need for there being better careers advice and development to allow doctors to restart career paths, retrain and diversify.[10] There are many reports of careers advice and guidance having been biased. Sometimes this is because the adviser is untrained and really giving informal careers advice about how to 'be like me'.[9] Doctors graduating from some medical schools in the UK are far more likely to opt for general practice, and the medical and surgical specialties, than those from others.[14] This difference is partly explained by some medical schools emphasising some specialties in ways that influence their graduates' career choices.

Individual doctors should be enabled to manage their careers more proactively with dependable careers information available on up-to-date websites, and improved access to impartial careers advice and guidance.

The need for careers advice and guidance in medical training and beyond

The NICEC report[8] recommended a model for provision of careers advice, much in line with calls from others.[8–11] The facilities these include are:

- careers education to be an integral part of the medical school curriculum
- high-quality careers information to be readily accessible and available about career and training options including national data on training places
- development of career management skills (self-assessment and career planning tools) as part of the curriculum in medical schools and postgraduate education
- proper training and support for doctors who provide informal and other careers advice
- trained career contacts and improved support networks; initiatives to improve the career support skills of experienced doctors, career mentoring programmes for overseas trained doctors and doctors from minority ethnic backgrounds
- careers advice to be signposted more clearly
- availability of impartial and expert advice; a network of advisers trained in career counselling with detailed knowledge of medical training
- national co-ordination of proposed sources of career development and support for doctors and medical students.

A pilot project of doctors in training emphasised the part that human resources personnel can play in helping to prepare doctors to secure a particular post in terms of curriculum vitae (CV) and interview skills, as well as potentially providing impartial and expert career counselling.[15] This echoed the experience of the *Don't Waste Doctors* initiative of the 1990s, where careers guidance outside the traditional medical hierarchy was created to give personal support and non-directive career counselling where needed.[12]

Career planning

Doctors need to:

- be aware that they should continually develop themselves throughout their careers
- take responsibility for managing their own learning and career development
- develop skills to learn from all their experiences.

Career planning can be structured as in the three stages of Box 1.1.

Box 1.1:   Checklist for a healthy career

- What do I *want* to do?
- What *can* I do?
- What am I *going* to do?

Careers information

Careers information gives the facts about the qualifications and experience needed for alternative career pathways and the opportunities that there are for career progression. This includes written and/or verbal information about the number and type of posts available at various levels in particular specialties and fields, and details of the qualifications and training necessary.[16]

Once a medical student or doctor knows what they want to do there are many sources of careers information. If they still don't know what they want to do, they may need careers advice or guidance to direct them to the careers information and opportunities that are available, or career counselling could help them to explore their strengths and discover different career and life options.

The national NHS Careers initiative in England provides much of the basic information about entry criteria and details of training for all type of careers in the health field. Paper and electronic information resources capture the individual experiences of health professionals describing their daily working lives, or look at the website of *NHS Professionals* (*see* Box 1.2) for more ideas.[17]

The key to good career planning is information gathering from people, books, and general observation. There are some good books that describe the wide variety of jobs and opportunities available to doctors, giving ideas about what else to try and how to branch out – into a career in journalism, sports medicine etc.[16,18–20]

You should be able to give, or signpost doctors to, information about:

- the qualifications and opportunities for all sorts of posts or alternative specialties
- educational opportunities: bursaries, grants, new and established degree courses
- non-health careers.

Box 1.2:   NHS Professionals www.nhsprofessionals.nhs.uk

NHS Professionals is a special health authority which is essentially a non-profit-making in-house staff agency for the NHS in England. It provides locum staff and keeps a register of their activity. The organisation manages temporary and flexible workers in the NHS, and supports these groups of staff, in an attempt to reduce their isolation.

Careers advice or guidance

Careers advice or guidance is personal and directive and provides advice within the context of the opportunities that are available. It is useful for those doctors who have not made a career decision, or are unaware of the best way of achieving their career goals.[16]

Such doctors might find it helpful to talk over where they are at with you or another careers adviser. This could be someone with a designated job in careers guidance, or it could be a mentor, a friend or colleague, an old tutor or the local continuing professional development (CPD) tutor. Someone providing careers advice or guidance should know about, and be able to provide, advice within the context of the opportunities that are available to the doctor.

Without adequate careers support they may remain ignorant of the options available, spend too much time in posts that are not ultimately relevant, and even be lost to the NHS altogether if they do not find the right niche.

As the person giving advice or guidance you should be well informed about the options and opportunities, and provide information or advice that is not biased. Trust managers may not give impartial advice to doctors about their career development if they wish to retain them in their current posts, or fill posts that fit with the trust's or practice's priorities. The quotes included in Box 1.3 reflect the lack of well-structured and informed careers advice those cited have received.

Box 1.3:   Lack of careers advice and guidance for doctors and medical students[9,15]

'Career advice usually happens after a chance conversation when you just start talking.'

'I need someone to invest in me as a person – someone who is interested in my existence.'

'Career advice is often perceived as something that anyone can do.'

'It's all word of mouth – it's who you know – everything is down to the individual.'

'One of the most daunting things of your PRHO [pre-registration house officer] year is suddenly having to put a CV together completely on your own.'

'Medical school is one of those funny things. You can go there for five years and you have not really got a clue about thinking about jobs, how to apply, where to apply.'

'I have not thoroughly researched what each [specialty] involves, just what you hear from word of mouth around the hospital really.'

Career counselling[16,21,22]

Career counselling is an intensive process requiring specialist skills. Career counselling is an umbrella term for the process of enabling somebody to evaluate their current situation and identify what steps are needed in order to change. It will usually include identification of a person's strengths and weaknesses in relation to their work options, and possibly bring in a variety of careers information.

The extent and type of help and support people need depends on their personal circumstances; career counselling may then be more appropriate than careers guidance. Career counselling has the potential to help health professionals and managers at all stages of their NHS careers, but may be particularly important for those thinking of returning to practice, people who are unhappy or dissatisfied with their careers, or doctors who want to discuss flexible career paths rather than long-term commitments.

Career counselling is a *process* and not an *event*. It involves the career counsellor being alongside someone, listening to them carefully and supporting them as they work through their problems. This process should enable people to recognise and utilise their own resources to manage career-related problems and make career decisions.

In most respects, career counselling is similar to any other kind of counselling in that it offers a framework for looking at problem situations and provides support to enable the person with the problem to undertake whatever changes they may decide to make. Successful career counselling will enable that person to identify the issues that need to be dealt with and mobilise the resources they need to improve matters. A well-trained career counsellor can help you to work out solutions to your difficulties, as described in Box 1.4.

Box 1.4:

Career counselling could help doctors to:

- think carefully about taking time out from their medical career
- re-evaluate their career choice and why they are considering a change
- re-assess whether they work part-time or full-time or retire early
- match their strengths to a career specialty or way of working that suits them – e.g. taking on more responsibility, or extending their skills (e.g. becoming a practitioner with special interest or trying a secondment to management).

People need career counselling when:

- they are dissatisfied with their current job or career prospects
- they seem unable to solve their career dilemma by themselves
- their thinking is clouded about their career and they need to talk things through with someone who is independent and non-judgemental
- they are not responding to the usual motivators at work
- they seem unaware of the consequences of their poor performance or behaviour at work
- they are engaging in self-deprecating behaviour at work
- they are unaware of their talents and strengths at work.

Career counselling allows the person to tell their story, then to start thinking about what would need to be in place for the situation to be improved, and finally to work out an action plan to deliver those changes. Career counselling involves matching the components of a job with a person's preferences, strengths and qualifications. The match between the choice of career and personality are very important and dictate personal preferences for the balances between work and leisure, work and income, degree of responsibility, type of work and extent of interaction with people.

The stages of career counselling are getting people to think through the following sequence of challenges:

- who am I and where am I now?
- how satisfied am I with my career and my life?
- what changes would I like to make?
- how do I make them happen?
- what do I do if I don't get what I want?

Any successful action plan needs a timescale and a description of what is possible in the short, medium and long-term. The outcome of career counselling should be *action.*

Finding a well-informed careers adviser or career counsellor

Careers advisers and career counsellors should be well informed, skilled and offer impartial help. Sometimes the same person is expected to be a mentor, educational supervisor, line manager and careers adviser or counsellor to one individual, and role conflicts can arise. If someone acting as a careers adviser or counsellor has line management authority, then the doctor concerned will be unlikely to trust in their independence. Worse still, they may act on their acquired insider knowledge on a future occasion if, for example, they are undertaking an appraisal or performance review of the doctor or giving them a reference for a new post.

Careers guidance or counselling might be provided by a mentor or coach. These two roles are distinct and bring specific attributes to a relationship.

Seeking a mentor[23-25]

A mentor relationship should be pretty much a one-way relationship where the mentor has the time and capacity to listen and help facilitate the person being mentored (the mentee) in making decisions about their career. The emphasis is on the mentor helping the mentee to develop their own thinking and find their own way, not on teaching the mentee new skills or acting as a patron to ease the mentee's career path by special favours. The mentor should be interested in people's development.

A mentor helps the person being mentored to realise their potential by acting as a trusted and experienced guide on personal, professional and educational matters. A mentor may agree learning and development objectives with a mentee and subsequently guide the mentee to address their educational and development needs, identify their strengths and weaknesses, explore options with them, act as a challenger, encourage reflection and provide motivation. The doctor's relationship with their mentor should be one of mutual trust and respect in a supportive yet challenging relationship where the mentor remains non-judgemental.

A common framework used for mentoring follows three stages:

1 *exploration*: when the mentor listens and prompts the mentee with questions
2 *new understanding*: when the mentor listens and challenges the mentee, recognises the strengths and weaknesses of the ideas, shares experiences, establishes priorities, identifies development needs, gives information and supportive feedback
3 *action planning*: encourages new ways of thinking, helps the mentee reach a solution, agree goals and decide action plans.

A coach could be what is needed[23,24]

A coach could offer more directive help to a doctor about their career, in the same way that a sports coach urges an athlete on. Coaches work through one-to-one conversations in person or by email or telephone.

A good coach will be a successful motivator, be very supportive, establish a good rapport with the doctor being coached, be able to give constructive feedback, and set clear objectives. The coach may be the doctor's manager or tutor, unless an external coach is being employed. The coach will stretch and challenge them and encourage them to solve problems and make changes. A good coach is analytical rather than critical, and is able to depersonalise the problems discussed in coaching sessions by focusing on facts, outcomes and performance rather than personality or style.

Coaching involves a combination of psychology, business and communication skills. It consists of a partnership between coach and 'client' to clarify the client's goals for work and life and plan how to achieve those goals. The interactive relationship enhances the doctor's potential and performance to a greater extent than seemed possible when functioning on their own. Coaching is sometimes confined to learning a specific skill for a future event such as a job interview or presentation at a conference. At other times coaching might be more centred on the doctor as a whole, to help them progress more quickly with their professional and career development. Every coaching situation is different, as each coach has their own particular style of working, and each client will have their individual circumstances and be at a particular point in their life.

A professional or 'executive' coach generally has a minimum of five years' experience as a coach and a professional qualification such as clinical psychology, occupational psychology, diploma in counselling, master practitioner in neurolinguistic programming or psychotherapy. Such an experienced coach will have expert knowledge of leadership and management behaviour, know about theory and practice of organisational behaviour and human psychology, be accredited to use personality profile testing and other personal assessment techniques, and have many interpersonal skills.

Coaching usually starts with an evaluation of the doctor's current effectiveness and their use of time and the nature of their priorities. The coach will encourage the doctor to reflect on how they might build on their strengths to change their current situation. They will enable the doctor to overcome often self-imposed limitations that are stopping them from progressing as far or as fast as they might otherwise do. Their developing self-awareness and insight should lead to lasting change.

Outcomes of coaching vary, depending on the circumstances of the person being coached – as explained in Box 1.5. He or she may tackle their job more effectively and enthusiastically having clearer objectives. They may reorganise or change their situation at work so that they perform better; or re-evaluate their career and decide to find a different job.

> **Box 1.5:**
>
> 'During the coaching people gradually connect with their true ambitions and identify what steps are needed to achieve them. They gain more control of their lives and feel less tossed about by events. The feedback we get later from clients confirms that this is truly the case.'[24]

A typical framework for a coaching session might be to:

- hear what's happened since last meeting
- agree the topics to work on
- agree what should be achieved by the end of the session
- agree priorities if there are too many issues
- undertake problem solving for each priority issue
- discuss what is the issue and why it is important
- discuss what has been tried already
- agree what would be an ideal state
- debate what's preventing the ideal state from happening now
- establish the extent to which they are preventing the ideal state from being achieved
- explore the options for resolving their problems
- discuss what skills are needed for their preferred option
- agree their strategy and target(s)
- select appropriate training methods
- make a realistic timetable for the training that both agree.

Flexible working

With the need to retain doctors of any age, the NHS has developed new schemes and ways to adapt jobs to match the needs or preferences of individual doctors. Some trusts are introducing more flexible working opportunities in an attempt to boost recruitment, retention, motivation and employee productivity. There are different approaches: shift swapping, annualised hours, part-time working, job sharing, a regular day off to compensate for hours worked outside normal working hours.

The current emphasis on flexible working practices mean that doctors can combine more than one post into a portfolio career balancing clinical, managerial or academic work.

Why doctors leave the profession

The main reasons that doctors leave the medical profession are that they feel that:

- they are not valued
- they are not supported
- they have an unacceptable work/life balance.[12,26]

In one study of doctors who had left practice, all were interested in returning to practice if the circumstances and support were right.[26] So, careers advice and guidance should be available for those doctors contemplating a return to medicine with parallel support from occupational health services, mentoring and educational updating and support. Such doctors need help and flexibility in designing their working patterns to achieve an improved work/life balance.

Almost three-quarters of doctors in the BMA cohort study either currently work less than full-time or would like to do so in the future.[10] Improving working conditions to enable improvement of working lives for doctors seems key to retaining doctors in the UK and to their staying in medicine.[27]

Career barriers[28]

A recent BMA survey has shown that not enough is being done to remove obstacles faced by some doctors that inhibit their career progression.[28] Many barriers are still prevalent within medicine today. These barriers to career progression play a part in some doctors' decision to leave the profession altogether.

There is much anecdotal evidence of racism in the NHS and that doctors from minority ethnic groups find it difficult to progress in their chosen career specialty. Greater proportions of doctors from minority ethnic groups are concentrated in staff and associate specialist grades.[29] Doctors who come to the UK with international medical qualifications lack information about career paths and opportunities. They are often frustrated by the costs and lengthy process of passing the International English Language Testing System (IELTS) and Professional and Linguistic Assessment Board (PLAB) examinations, and subsequent difficulties of getting clinical attachments and first jobs. They are confused by which posts are and are not training posts. Many GPs from minority ethnic groups practise in deprived communities.

Doctors with disabilities or chronic illness face many difficulties.[30] They are often stigmatised. They encounter inflexible working patterns, poor cover arrangements, little allowance in training or working for their health needs, ill-prepared colleagues who make the doctor feel guilty about the way their disability or illness impacts on their work.

The distribution of men and women doctors through the career grades is disproportionate, and women doctors are under-represented in senior career grades. Sexist attitudes, a lack of flexibility and work–life imbalance of some specialties were blamed as causative factors.[28]

The BMA report relayed homophobic experiences and fear of discrimination by some lesbian, gay and bisexual doctors.

Doctors considering an academic career may be deterred by financial disincentives, the lack of a career structure and perceived clinical deskilling which is seen as a threat to resuming clinical responsibility. There are concerns that the recruitment and retention crisis in academic medicine will result in there being too few medical academics to teach the increasing numbers of medical students and doctors in their foundation years. Solutions such as seed corn funding to kickstart research, career pathways, more flexible working arrangements, salary equivalence with clinical posts, and mentoring are sought.[31,32]

We need to establish a generally enabling environment in the NHS for doctors and all the rest of the workforce, as proposed by all the organisations whose reports are cited here, as in Box 1.6.[1,2,7,8,10,28]

> **Box 1.6:**
>
> 'Creating an environment in which doctors are able to restart career paths, retrain and diversify without attracting criticism or detriment to their career is vital to ensuring high morale and motivation among junior doctors. This needs to be accompanied by better career advice and development and arrangements for re-entry after career breaks. Incentives designed to improve the working lives of doctors, value their professional contribution and support the continued development of their educational and training needs are crucial if the flow of doctors seeking a better life outside of the health service is to be stemmed.'[10]

Retaining doctors and encouraging doctors to return to practice

There are several initiatives designed to help retain or recruit doctors returning to work in the NHS. These are:

* the Flexible Career Scheme (FCS) for doctors of all grades in hospital, and GPs. It is for doctors who want to work less than 50% of full-time and at least 20% time. It may suit doctors at any stage of their career; for example, while looking after dependants, facilitating a doctor's return to practice, for doctors who are semi-retired, those wanting to retire from their regular job and return with different responsibilities. The FCS provides clinical and educational supervision, funding towards professional expenses and protected time for education. Doctors can work within the FCS for up to 3 years
* the Retainer Scheme for GPs wanting to work up to four half-days per week and at least half a day per week. There is clinical and educational supervision, and protected educational time, and contribution to professional expenses. The scheme normally lasts up to 5 years but can be extended for longer
* the Returner Scheme for GPs or hospital doctors is for doctors who have had a substantial career break (more than 12 months). The salary of the doctor is fixed at the level of when they last worked in the NHS. Refresher training in clinical, technology or management skills is individualised to the doctor's needs as determined by an initial assessment arranged by the deanery. The doctor can remain on the returner scheme for 6 months full-time, or 12 months part-time; and take up to six weeks study leave. The returner doctor may progress to the FCS or a substantive post.

NHS Professionals and the local deanery are the contacts for any of these schemes.[17,33,34] The Royal Colleges can offer support and advice (*see* Appendix 2).[35]

The *Improving Working Lives for Doctors* standard sets a model of good human resources practice against which NHS employers and their staff can measure their organisation's human resources (HR) management.[34] One standard that is particularly relevant to retaining doctors is the requirement for NHS employers to 'provide personal and professional development and training opportunities that are accessible and open to all staff irrespective of their working patterns'. The *Improving Working Lives* initiative should help all doctors to work more flexibly.[34] This will be particularly important for doctors with disabilities or chronic ill-health.[36]

Although progress is being made in encouraging doctors to complete and maintain personal development plans (PDPs) as part of the appraisal process, there should be more focus on specific professional or career development to encourage doctors and others to remain working in the NHS (*see* Chapter 7).

References

1   Binding C and Sowden D (2004) *Making Sense of the Medical Career Maze – a UK consultation document and proposal for implementation in Trent.* Trent Postgraduate Deanery, University of Nottingham, Nottingham.

2   Modernising Medical Careers Working Group for Career Management (2005) *Career Management: an approach for medical schools, deaneries, royal colleges and trusts.* The Stationery Office, London.

3   Department of Health (2005) *Hospital, Public Health Medicine and Community Health Services Medical and Dental Staff in England: 1994–2004.* Department of Health, London.

4   Department of Health (2004) *General and Personal Medical Services Statistics, Medical and Dental Workforce Census.* Department of Health, London.

5   MacDonald R (ed) (2004) *Overseas Doctors: sink or swim? Career focus information booklet.* BMJcareers supplement. www.bmjcareers.com (accessed 8 August 2005).

6   Department of Health (2003) *NHS International Medical Recruitment: case studies.* NHS Careers, Department of Health, London.

7   Department of Health (2004) *Modernising Medical Careers – the next steps. The future shape of foundation, specialist and general practice training programmes.* Department of Health, London.

8   The National Institute for Careers Education and Counselling (NICEC) (2003) *Informing Choices.* NICEC, Careers Research and Advisory Centre (CRAC), London.

9   Chambers R (1997) *Need for Careers Counselling for General Practice in the West Midlands Region.* Staffordshire University, Stoke-on-Trent.

10   British Medical Association (2004) *BMA Cohort Study of 1995 Medical Graduates. Ninth report.* Health Policy and Economic Research Unit, BMA, London.

11   British Medical Association (2003) *Sign-posting Medical Careers for Doctors.* Board of Medical Education, BMA, London.

12   Harvey J, Davison H, Winsland J et al. (1998) *Don't Waste Doctors. A report on wastage, recruitment and retention of doctors in the north west.* NHS Executive, Manchester.

13   Thornett A, Cobb S, Chambers R and Mohanna K (2005) Accessing careers support in primary care. *Education for Primary Care.* **16:** 66–73.

14   Goldacre MJ, Turner G and Lambert T (2004) Variation by medical school in career choices of UK graduates of 1999 and 2000. *Medical Education.* **38:** 249–58.

15   Bullock A, Field S, Burke S et al. (2004) *Careers Advice for Junior Doctors.* University of Birmingham, Birmingham.

16   Chambers R, Mohanna K and Field S (2000) *Opportunities and Options in Medical Careers.* Radcliffe Medical Press, Oxford.

17   NHS Professionals. Hotline +44 (0)845 60 60 345. www.nhsprofessionals.nhs.uk (accessed 8 August 2005).

18 Ward C and Eccles S (2001) *So You Want to be a Brain Surgeon?* (2e). Oxford University Press, Oxford.

19 Aquino P and Jones P (2004) *Career Options in General Practice*. Radcliffe Publishing, Oxford.

20 Baker M and Chambers R (2000) *A Guide to General Practice Careers*. Royal College of General Practitioners, London.

21 Rogers C (1999) *Client Centred Therapy*. Constable, London.

22 Egan G (1990) *The Skilled Helper* (6e). Brooks Cole Publishing Co, New York.

23 Mohanna K, Wall D and Chambers R (2004) *Teaching Made Easy* (2e). Radcliffe Medical Press, Oxford.

24 Parsloe E and Wray M (2003) *Coaching and Mentoring*. Kogan Page, London.

25 Bayley H, Chambers R and Donovan C (2004) *The Good Mentoring Toolkit for Healthcare*. Radcliffe Publishing, Oxford.

26 British Medical Association (2004) *Why do Doctors Leave the Profession?* Health Policy and Economic Research Unit, BMA, London.

27 Moss PJ, Lambert TW, Goldacre MJ and Lee P (2004) Reasons for considering leaving UK medicine: questionnaire study of junior doctors' comments. *British Medical Journal*. **329:** 1263–5.

28 British Medical Association (2004) *Career Barriers in Medicine: doctors' experiences*. British Medical Association, London.

29 MacDonald R (2004) *Non-standard Grade (Trust) Doctors: The Truth. Career focus information guide*. BMJcareers supplement. www.bmjcareers.com

30 MacDonald R (2004) *Training and Working with Disabilities*. Career focus information guide. BMJcareers supplement. www.bmjcareers.com (accessed 8 August 2005).

31 British Medical Association (2004) *Medical Academic Career Intentions*. Health Policy and Economic Unit, British Medical Association, London.

32 Academic Careers Sub-committee of Modernising Medical Careers and the UK Clinical Research Collaboration (2005) *Medically and Dentally Qualified Academic Staff: recommendations for training the researchers and educators of the future*. MMC, London.

33 www.gprecruitment.org.uk (accessed 8 August 2005).

34 Department of Health (2002) *Improving Working Lives for Doctors*. Department of Health, London.

35 Royal College of General Practitioners (2005) *A Career in General Practice: education, training and professional development*. RCGP Information Sheet. Royal College of General Practitioners, London.

36 Department of Health (2004) *Sharing the Challenge, Sharing the Benefits. Equality and diversity in the medical workforce*. Department of Health, London.

2

What *Modernising Medical Careers* means for doctors

Steve Field

This chapter draws heavily on the UK Careers Management Strategy written by members of the Careers Management Working Group of the MMC Advisory Board, chaired by Steve Field. We give special thanks to Charlene Binding, Guidance and Support Associate, Trent Postgraduate Deanery, and Dr Stuart Carrney, specialist registrar in psychiatry, and training adviser to the MMC team.

The four UK Departments of Health launched their ambitious UK-wide approach to the delivery of career management in summer 2005 as part of their *Modernising Medical Careers* (MMC) agenda. The strategy focused on a career management model that was developed by the working group of the MMC Advisory Board with the expert guidance of Charlene Binding, Guidance and Support Associate in the Trent Postgraduate Deanery. The full strategy document can be accessed on the *Modernising Medical Careers* website.[1]

The career management strategy presents deans of medical schools and postgraduate deans across the UK with the challenge to provide a proactive and educational approach to career management in their localities, to replace the old informal, patchy and unregulated system.

The strategy covers the continuum of medical careers, from before starting university, through selection to medical school, undergraduate and postgraduate training through to that of retiring doctors. It also seeks to respond to students and doctors where there may be cause for concern, and to help students and doctors who have few ideas about which career may suit them.

The idea is to encourage the independence of the individual doctor in making an informed career choice, through facilitation and support. It recognises that career aspirations and choices must be aligned with actual service need and what employers require of their workforce. The strategy takes into account the impact that medical and technological advances can have on students' and doctors' career opportunities and hopes. For example it has become clear that the NHS is training too many cardiothoracic surgeons for the future needs of the service, because of changes in medical and surgical treatments, the rise of angioplasty, the use of stents and the increasing amount of their work taken on by cardiologists and interventional radiologists. Deans have had to counsel trainees that there may be insufficient consultant posts for them when they complete their training programmes, and have helped facilitate their transfer into other specialties' training programmes. Career management, therefore, must be flexible to ensure that advice and support is directed at the needs of individual doctors within the context of the needs of the NHS.

The career management system should offer a range of processes, activities and initiatives in the context of continued reflective practice, transparency and continuous evaluation of the range of activities. The career management model asserts the following principles:

- career decision making is a lifetime continuum rather than an event which 'happens' in the early years of a doctor's career or when career difficulties or crises are faced
- the career support needs of some target groups have a greater priority (e.g. doctors in foundation years 1 and 2 making significant career choices early in their careers, international medical graduates entering the UK)
- career management services are an essential feature of the training and development a doctor should expect from the deanery or trust training and/or employing them
- the deanery should enable individual doctors, strategic health authorities (SHAs) and employing trusts, to realise the benefits of accessible and available career management services. This includes enabling individuals to utilise careers information, advice and guidance to gain insight into the careers for which they are suited and to examine a range of careers opportunities which may be available to them
- career management services should support informed careers choice and be primarily driven by the needs of the individual doctor, while closely aligning these with medical service demands and needs
- career support services should cater for all individuals whatever their circumstances, and be able to handle complex situations including doctors about whom there is concern or who have personal difficulties
- those educators and others providing careers support should have the dedicated time to fulfil their role effectively, both in terms of their own preparation and training and the actual delivery of career management services.

The MMC career management delivery model

The strategy acknowledges the number of local initiatives and national providers of careers information that already exist, but requests a more co-ordinated delivery which is inclusive and builds on existing good practice. It offers the career management delivery model as a focus for discussion between each postgraduate deanery, working in conjunction with their local community and medical schools, workforce development directorates of strategic health authorities and NHS trusts – as to how career management delivery can be addressed (*see* Figure 2.1).

The model seeks to address the needs of the following groups along the continuum of a doctor's career:

- school children and school leavers contemplating a medical career
- university and medical school graduates
- foundation doctors
- senior clinicians' continuing professional development needs
- specific groups such as those undertaking part-time or flexible careers
- international medical graduates who are working or want to work in the UK
- those contemplating retirement and beyond.

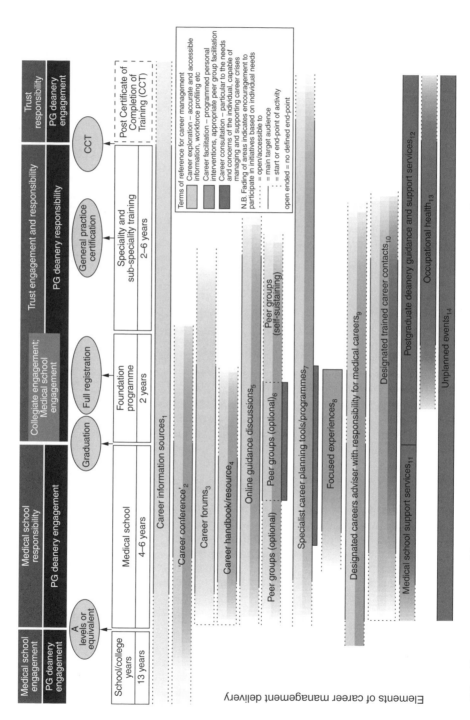

Figure 2.1: Career management delivery model of the *Modernising Medical Careers* initiative for the UK.[1]

Within those groups there may be students and doctors who give cause for concern about their practice, some who are experiencing some kind of 'career crisis', others who have no idea for which career they may be best suited, or some who are doing well in their careers but are not maximising their skills and aptitudes in their current job.

Delivery aspects: explanations of elements of the model

The career management model is divided into 14 main elements of delivery (*see* the corresponding heading and annotated number within Figure 2.1). There should be a suggested lead for each of the 14 elements from the key organisations involved, who can proactively contribute and support each element of career management delivery.

In the case of the delivery and implementation of career management initiatives during Foundation Programme Training, the following section should be read in conjunction with *Modernising Medical Careers' Operational Framework for Foundation Programmes.*[2]

1 Career information sources – at local and national levels

The availability of reliable, up-to-date information is essential. Local information supported by deanery networks should assist prospective medical trainees in making more informed choices about their prospective career. Deaneries have a central role in bringing together the different sources of information. Many deaneries already use their websites to provide information for their trainees with links to Royal Colleges and specialist societies, universities, local employing trusts and other key stake-holders. A survey of deaneries by Eaton in 2004 demonstrated that five deaneries specifically mentioned the development of web-based deanery career information (West Midlands; Northern; Trent; Leicestershire, Northamptonshire and Rutland (LNR); and London).[3] The West Midlands Deanery website, with careers information established for many years, includes competition ratios for all specialties.[4] Following the publication of the national guidelines, other deaneries have begun to develop their own web resources. The information that will be made available by deaneries will include:

- the variety of jobs available by location across the deanery area
- the qualifications and training requirements for different medical careers
- personal perspectives of posts (e.g. case studies, vignettes, video clips)
- deanery and national competition ratios for programmes
- the annual number of applications for training programmes and appointments
- illustrative career paths.

Local information should be supplemented by national resources. Deanery websites will be linked to Royal College and specialist society websites. There will also eventually be national medical career resources developed by the four devolved national health services as part of the *Modernising Medical Careers* agenda. In England, a 'one stop national shop' is being planned by NHS Careers in partnership with the MMC working group. NHS Careers already provides a helpline, a web-based information service which offers information on careers across the NHS, including some information on medical careers, but it has been mainly aimed at non-medical staff groups, prospective new entrants to the NHS, while also providing a service advertising some job vacancies. It is hoped that the helpline service will be expanded and that it will become the central focus of careers information for doctors working in partnership with deaneries to ensure that information is kept up to date.

2 Career conference or fair

This would usually be an annual event, open to medical students and junior doctors organised by, or on behalf of, deaneries in partnership with local medical schools, strategic health authorities, trusts and other stakeholders. The career conference aims at enabling participants to learn more about potential career choices. It should include presentations on key themes of the day, e.g. *Modernising Medical Careers*, the Postgraduate Medical Education and Training Board or a new training programme, but also include workshops targeted at the development of general skills such as self-awareness and overall career management skills development. Opportunities to learn more about how to write CVs, apply for training programmes and improve interview skills are appropriate workshops run as part of the conference programme.

A very successful example of such a conference is the annual 'BMJ Career Fair' held in London and more recently in Scotland. Further collaborations between deaneries and the *British Medical Journal* (*BMJ*) include more BMJ Career Fairs to be held in the Midlands and in the North of England.

3 Career forums

A career forum is a key local event aimed at senior medical students, junior doctors and more established doctors. A career forum provides an ideal opportunity for trainees in the Foundation Programme training, and for those entering or re-entering medical training or wishing to take a career break to further their career planning and development. They also represent useful opportunities to make contacts, exchange career ideas, and begin to build relevant career networks with other colleagues.

The career forum should complement the larger careers conference and ideally be held more frequently with different foci covering the main specialties. It could also focus on specific topics such as flexible training and academic careers.

The West Midlands Deanery holds career forums at their deanery offices covering specific needs of international medical graduates, refugees and those wishing to train flexibly. They plan to extend the system of monthly career forums to cover different specialty areas, e.g. medical specialties, surgical specialties, general practice and flexible careers etc. They are delivered in partnership with the local medical schools and NHS trusts and are to be held in venues across the region. The format is one of short presentations on the specialty area, followed by time for group and individual discussions.

4 Career handbook

Some medical schools and postgraduate deaneries have developed local careers handbooks – a good example of an accessible and comprehensive guide being the

Nottingham/Trent Deanery handbook.[5] These supply information relevant to the local medical school or deanery area, and usually complement local web-based information. They outline main points of contact for career support networks, e.g. clear signposting of mentors, career coaches, educational supervisors etc.

While no comprehensive national career resources exist that provide unbiased information across specialties or along the continuum of a doctor's career, information on individual specialties is available from Royal Colleges and specialist societies. The main source of up-to-date written information is the BMJ Careers Focus which provides careers information and advice for medical students and doctors. It also advertises job opportunities and courses, and provides advice for overseas doctors and for disabled doctors.

5 Online careers guidance discussions

Online career initiatives are being developed by the NHS, Royal Colleges, deaneries and commercial providers. In addition to being information sources, they may include e-guidance initiatives and online career discussions.

E-guidance initiatives provide an optional means of accessing potentially in-depth careers guidance from a range of people who have been prepared adequately for this role (whether medical, non-medical or other health professional). Online career discussions are web based, where appropriately skilled, trained and professionally supported individuals mediate to keep topics up to date and help build wider networks with contributing individuals. The maintenance of a local online career resource is a logical adjunct to the provision of local careers information highlighted above. Medical Forum provides personalised careers guidance, and opportunities for professional growth and personal development for medical and dental professionals.[6] It is hoped that NHS Careers will develop its information service to include an e-guidance and discussion facility.

Other initiatives include the BMJCareers 'Advice Zone' which maintains a growing database of career queries and the BMJCareers 'Jobscore' initiative (*see* page 25).[7,8] Advice can also be obtained from Royal Colleges and deanery websites, while NHS Professionals provides guidance on flexible careers[9] and the Medical Women's Federation offers members advice and support in their careers.[10]

6 Peer group activities

Peer group activities are a key component of the career management model. They are particularly suited to the medical school and Foundation Programme years. Medical students should be actively encouraged to attend activities that would typically be time limited over a number of weeks or months during the undergraduate years. It is intended that the environment would be supportive, so that participants could discuss and learn from their thoughts about their future career, and to develop and monitor individual and group career action plans. The groups should ideally be a proper part of an undergraduate curriculum and begin soon after the student starts at medical school.

In addition to being a forum for discussion, independent and facilitated career planning activities and career exploration tools could be used to help students and junior doctors explore ways of aligning their aptitudes, strengths and career interests, e.g. facilitated use and interpretation of the medical career software package: The

Specialty Choice Inventory – Sci45[11,12] – appropriate tailoring of other career exploration tools and programmes including Myers Briggs preference profiling[13] or comparable tools are good examples. In addition, practical aspects of developing employability skills, such as application processes, CV and interview technique could be usefully addressed at the same time.

During the latter years of medical school, peer groups will become more focused on the challenge 'where am I going and why?' in career planning and thinking. Encouragement and support from an experienced and trained facilitator is essential; this will be an appropriately trained tutor, coach or mentor, and not necessarily a doctor.

These peer group discussions and activities will help medical students focus on their desired career pathways now that decision making will be much earlier in their career because of the changes in training programmes as a result of *Modernising Medical Careers*. Medical students should be able to demonstrate their rationale for their particular career interests by the time of graduation, and show evidence of how they have made initial future career plans.

During the Foundation Programme years, peer development groups should continue to be offered and placements arranged to help the doctor refine or confirm their career intentions prior to applying for a specialist or general practice training programme.

7 Specialist career planning tools or programmes

Specialist career planning tools and programmes should be available for medical students and junior doctors locally and nationally – from medical schools, postgraduate deaneries and trusts in order to promote enhanced career and life insights, either as part of peer group work or in other formats (e.g. e-guidance). They should be expertly facilitated so that they contribute to the developmental processes of doctors' lifelong learning and career development. Tools such as Sci45 have already been used by thousands of students and junior doctors, but facilitation is vital.[11,12] This should be provided by either an in-depth one-to-one encounter, or by peer group conversations with appropriately skilled and trained career management professionals, and include objective feedback on the student's or doctor's career preference.

8 Focused experiences

The GMC has been a strong advocate of special study modules (SSMs) and electives during medical school. These provide ideal opportunities to taste different career opportunities that students do not usually encounter during their undergraduate years. These may be in a clinical specialty such as radiology or public health, or in a subject such as academic medicine, management, journalism, or medical politics. The Foundation Programme should also offer opportunities for the trainee to attend clinics, inner city or rural training practices, or pursue a research agenda.

9 Designated careers advisers

In 2005, the Department of Health of England provided significant financial resources to employ a dedicated team of career advisers in each deanery as part of the MMC

Management Strategy. The other home countries also promised to support the strategy.

The 'ring-fenced' investment is aimed at providing a career adviser in every foundation school to act as a co-ordinator of careers activities in each locality. They should improve communication and co-ordinate the delivery of the career management model locally as a partnership between the deanery, medical schools, university career services and NHS trusts. While the majority of work will be focused on developing local networks, the career adviser will also liaise closely with other deaneries and national resources, e.g. NHS Careers and Royal Colleges, to develop a comprehensive service for local medical students and junior doctors.

10 Designated trained career contacts

This element of the model emphasises the provision of more targeted one-to-one, online or peer group initiatives at local and national levels. The following multi-professional groups form an essential feature of such provision:

- appropriately qualified doctors: e.g. Royal College tutors or advisers, educational and clinical supervisors, tutors, mentors, associate deans with particular specialty career interests, and/or who represent shortage specialties and academic careers
- clinical staff: e.g. nursing and allied health professionals who may have close working contact with undergraduate medical students and junior doctors
- non-medical professionals: e.g. qualified careers advisers, experienced facilitators, HR representatives, postgraduate education centre managers and staff, those in pastoral support roles etc.

As with the role of the career adviser, designated trained career contacts can help to make appropriate 'career readiness' assessments with medical undergraduates and trainees.

All those who have undertaken a more formalised career support role should have protected time to deliver such provision. This could be usefully underpinned by a generic model of practice to promote consistency and continuity between providers, whether regionally or nationally.

11 Medical school support services

Medical schools already offer a range of services for their students, but they vary between schools across the country. The new designated careers advisers will support the medical schools and ensure that good practice is disseminated. Medical school support services are usually available by self-referral, and include facilitated provision of student support and guidance. In future they will connect with other aspects of career management outlined in the model, i.e. peer groups, one-to-one advice, online initiatives etc, and in particular with the postgraduate deanery.

12 Postgraduate deanery guidance and support services

All postgraduate deaneries have services that support medical trainees who are in difficulty. Some also have confidential services for doctors that include the opportunity to discuss personal health issues.

The West Midlands Deanery, for example, co-ordinates a service to support doctors in difficulty who are either self-referred, referred by educational supervisors or via the record of in-training assessment (RITA) process, or referred by the National Clinical Assessment Service (NCAS), GMC or NHS trusts. The deanery also funds an externally delivered confidential counselling service called 'Contact', for doctors who may be stressed or wish to discuss confidential health issues. The deanery has trained a number of deanery educators at Staffordshire University in order to expand the service to offer targeted career consultations and realistic feedback on career concerns. The expanded service will liaise closely with other key stakeholders in doctors' careers, including Royal Colleges, the GMC, the BMA, NHS Professionals and employing NHS trusts etc.

13 Occupational health and occupational psychology

Part of the national careers strategy that will be difficult for individual postgraduate deaneries to deliver is access to a suitably trained occupational psychologist to respond to doctors with specific career needs (using suitable avenues for referral). While all deaneries will be able to access occupational health advice, occupational psychologists will only occasionally be needed for those doctors who are unable to pursue a particular career option, for example as a result of a failure to make adequate educational progress, or due to a disability or other specific factors. This specialised service may be shared between deaneries to cover the whole of the UK; the *Modernising Medical Careers* working group are investigating this possibility.

14 Unplanned events

More common than the planned meeting or intervention is the chance conversation, experience or event that can lead an individual student or doctor to pursue or deviate from a particular career path. With more structured career management, students and doctors will be encouraged to be more proactive in their career planning, and focus their training on their ultimate career goal. Those working in medical schools and deaneries will, therefore, need to be better equipped to cope with the more knowledgeable medical student or trainee and be able to help direct them into the appropriate part of the new system.

Chapter 10 discusses an approach you might take as a deanery, SHA, trust or practice to agree and implement a careers strategy based on this career management model.

References

1   www.mmc.nhs.uk (accessed 8 August 2005).

2   Modernising Medical Careers Working Group for Career Management (2005) *Career Management: an approach for medical schools, deaneries, royal colleges and trusts.* The Stationery Office, London.

3   Eaton J (2004) *Career Management Support for Trainees – a survey of English deaneries.* Committee of Postgraduate Medical Deans (COPMeD), London.

4   The West Midlands Deanery website. www.wmdeanery.org

5   Department of Health (2005) *Operational Guide to Foundation Programmes (The Purple Guide)*. Department of Health, London.

6   www.medicalforum.com (accessed 8 August 2005).

7   www.bmjcareers.com (accessed 8 August 2005).

8   MacDonald R (2004) Rating jobs with JobScore. *BMJ Careers*. **13 November:** 200–21. www.bmjcareers.com/jobscore (accessed 8 August 2005).

9   www.nhsprofessionals.nhs.uk (accessed 8 August 2005).

10   www.medicalwomensfederation.org.uk (accessed 8 August 2005).

11   Gale R and Grant J (2001) *Sci45 The Specialty Choice Inventory. Computer based careers advice for doctors in training.* Open University for Education in Medicine, Milton Keynes.

12   Gale R and Grant J (2002) Sci45: the development of a specialty choice inventory. *Medical Education.* **36:** 659–66.

13   Briggs Myers I and Briggs B (1995) *Gifts Differing – understanding personality type.* Davies-Black, California.

3

What careers information should you make available to doctors?

Andrew Thornett

The scope of careers information that you should make available to doctors is summarised in Box 3.1. It includes the provision of written and/or verbal information about career opportunities, including the number and type of posts available at a particular level and in a particular specialty, and details of the qualifications and training necessary. It also includes information on where to go to access more intensive support options.

Box 3.1: Scope of provision of careers information[1]

Aspect 1: Range of career options
Description: knows where information about the range of options in medical careers can be found. (Depth of knowledge ranges from general awareness to detailed knowledge of *sources of* information for all specialties, parallel careers, allied non-health posts.)

Aspect 2: Qualifications, training and experience for various health careers
Description: knows range of options in medical careers for NHS workforce in primary care settings – including qualifications, training and experience needed, number and type of posts available at various levels. (Depth of knowledge ranges from general awareness to detailed knowledge of all specialties, parallel careers, allied non-health posts.)

Aspect 3: Current regulations relating to doctors in training and their qualifications
Description: knows current regulations relating to doctors in training and their gaining of qualifications. (Depth of knowledge ranges from general awareness to accurate details of regulations for doctors who have trained overseas, have taken a prolonged career break, have taken unusual career routes and want to (re-) enter a particular specialty.)

> **Aspect 4: Personal perspectives of career specialties**
> *Description*: Knows where individuals requiring personal careers information can find help from an experienced person in type of post. (Depth of knowledge ranges from general awareness to details/backgrounds of wide range of post-holders.)

In the past, careers information has been too general and rarely kept as an updated resource. Doctors today regard the provision of personalised information and advice as a key component of high-quality careers support. They are keen to receive information and advice that is specific to their individual professional needs, and takes account of their family and personal situations.

Many doctors have a clear idea of the career options open to them and simply want relevant information to help them to choose between these options. Others have access to informal support networks that they trust and similarly wish only to obtain up-to-date information from you. Only a small number will require referral for more in-depth careers guidance.

Be prepared with good careers information

As someone giving careers information, whether you are a peer adviser, appraiser or part of more formal careers support services, you should have access to up-to-date information about the careers options likely to be of most interest to those seeking your help. You need to be aware of the implications for doctors' careers of government policies and guidance, and should have copies of example hospital and general practice contracts available. You need access to databases of local career opportunities, including salaried and principal posts in general practice, hospital posts at all grades, and opportunities to develop additional roles as part of a doctor's portfolio career. Be aware of what training and funding are available to allow doctors to make career changes if they require it. Be able to offer contact details if they are keen to seek more intensive career guidance or counselling.

You should be confident that your knowledge remains current and up to date. Attending careers fairs, staying in close contact with key players in your local region to ensure that your knowledge of opportunities is complete, and regular scanning of the deanery website and other reliable internet sites should all help to keep you updated.

Online systems such as www.bmjcareers.com/advicezone offer an enquiry service, and previously posed questions and their answers are available for all to read. Doctors can type in a search phrase and the system will bring up questions previously asked on the issue. The answers given are specific to the original question, but doctors can extrapolate information for their own situation, to help in their decision-making.

JobScore (www.bmjcareers.com/jobscore) is a free online medical careers service created by doctors for doctors. It is an 'evidence-based job hunting' system to help doctors make informed job choices from a peer-reviewed database on hospital jobs throughout the UK. It provides peer reviews of medical jobs submitted by doctors who have recently worked in them. It covers all specialties at all grades in all hospitals throughout the UK. Those searching the site have to contribute at least one report of a post they have recently held.

What information about careers should you be able to provide for doctors as their supervisor, tutor, trainer, appraiser?

Doctors are keen to have information that is placed in the context of the complexities and political realities of working in the NHS. They want it to be up to date to reflect the changing job situation in the UK, including new contractual arrangements in both primary and secondary care, new opportunities for ways of working, increased availability of salaried posts, part-time positions and work outside general practice or hospital.

Medical students and doctors want careers information that takes account of their personal as well as their professional needs, regardless of their age, sex, or clinical experience. As an experienced professional, you are particularly well placed to develop and deliver such information. There are some differences between the needs and characteristics of groups of doctors.

Medical students and newly qualified doctors

Medical students and newly qualified doctors are keen to receive summary information on a large range of possible career options available, obtaining high-quality information on the first steps they should take in becoming a specialist. They will want more detailed information on the requirements they need to fulfil to progress in the smaller number of career paths that particularly interest them, as in Box 3.2 and Box 3.3. This may involve general advice on the suitability of different types of applicant for a particular job, the pros and cons of taking up alternative employment options, and the respective competition ratios (the numbers of applicants applying for positions in each specialty against the number of positions available). Examples of competition ratios for medical specialties are given at www.wmdeanery.org/careerguide/guide/31.htm. Medical students and newly qualified doctors will be keen to return to this database from time to time to explore individual options further.

Box 3.2:   How you might respond to a frequently asked question (FAQ):*
What qualifications or experience are needed to follow a particular career path?

The information you provide should describe the range of doctors who have taken up this option in the past. Are there any minimal experiential requirements? If so, in what sphere of practice and for how long? What sort of training will be provided as part of the post? What other skills and experience could a doctor interested in such a position bring with them to improve their chances of pursuing this career path? Many medical positions require particularly high levels of commitment. Would it be advantageous to have a particular interest in the area in question?

Do not forget to mention the financial opportunities and likely effects on family life if the doctor took up this position, as these may be important factors in the decision about a career path for many doctors.

* This FAQ and others in this chapter have been adapted from www.bmjcareers.com/advicezone and other sources.

Box 3.3:   How you might respond to a specific FAQ: What does the discipline of particular subject area cover?

This type of question is the bread and butter of careers information packs about particular specialties, which traditionally provide general information on career options and requirements for entry. Ensure that you think broadly and cover all the areas in which those who will be reading your literature or hearing you speak or discussing their situation in a one-to-one arrangement will be interested.

Newly qualified doctors may be anxious about the implications for their future careers of decisions they make now. The ethos of medicine is to understand disease in detail in order to treat it, and many of these doctors would like to address their careers in the same way, seeking out in-depth knowledge of the career options and then the pros and cons of each option open to them. Do not forget to mention possibilities for portfolio careers and to include salaried as well as GP partnership options in general practice,[2] although at this stage most doctors are mainly concerned with establishing themselves in a specialty.

Established doctors

For the majority of doctors established in their careers in general practice or hospital medicine, the emphasis is upon obtaining information about additional roles that could improve their job satisfaction and enjoyment in working, or on preparing for retirement (*see* page 11 to read about the flexible careers scheme). The information you give should be broad and demonstrate a range of flexible options that allow them to continue to work at their main job. Detailed advice and contact details of relevant bodies should be readily available.

For other doctors who are dissatisfied with their current roles or seeking a change because they are bored or have developed a disability for instance, the need is for information on what alternative career options are open to them. This may include a change of specialty, a change of employer or GP partnership, a reduction or change in the pattern of work they do, or retraining as in Box 3.4. For these doctors, the emphasis is upon improving the quality of their life, and careers information should include aspects of the career options that impact directly upon their personal and professional wants and needs.[3] Get them to consider how the alternative career path will affect the time they have to spend with their family. This group may have significant financial commitments and they will be particularly interested in the financial remuneration each career option provides, and its effect on future financial planning. Remember to signpost links to information on pensions, housing and house prices if the option includes moving area, leisure facilities, schools and school fees, and average cost of living in various localities.

> **Box 3.4:** How you might respond to a specific FAQ: Request for information on retraining in a different discipline or practice area
>
> Exact information and advice depends upon the medical discipline that the doctor would like to pursue and their previous experience. In many cases a useful response will require in-depth careers advice or counselling. Think broadly and cover the range of career options. Although particular paths may not be open to someone who comes from a different specialty, other options may be. In some cases, training in advance of application is required, but in others it is provided on the job.[4]

Careers information can be particularly reassuring to a doctor in this position, increasing his or her confidence that an acceptable and enjoyable alternative career path or job does exist for them. In itself, this will encourage them to continue to seek further information and, where appropriate, take up careers advice and/or career counselling.

One particular mistake that is easy to make is to assume that doctors in their mid-career are knowledgeable and experienced at career planning and know where to access careers information. Many GPs, for instance, joined a partnership straight after GP training, or established consultants may have had a straightforward career track for many years. It may have been many years since they last sought out careers information. Many alternative career options will have changed significantly and new options will be available – as a result established doctors may be less knowledge-able than many newly qualified doctors, and are likely to have much more significant family and social ties that limit their flexibility.

Career change for these doctors is often a complex process requiring careful planning and thought. A portfolio of different roles need to be carefully fitted together to ensure that the doctor can meet his or her commitments on an ongoing basis and continue to enjoy the benefits of diversifying their career. Additional roles may include diversification from traditional clinical work through managerial or political roles, teaching or research. The careers information you provide should include sources of training and funding to undertake these potential new roles, and not just focus on the roles themselves.

Doctors taking career breaks

Some training schemes and disciplines are more understanding than others about career breaks, and your careers information should give a broad indication of the differences in attitudes between disciplines, *see* Box 3.5.

> **Box 3.5:** How you might respond to a specific FAQ: I would like to take a break from medicine. What effect will this have on my career progression?
>
> The reason for the career break is probably more important than the break itself in terms of its effect on a doctor's career progression after returning to work. Many interviewers will ask specifically about gaps in service on CVs, seeking reassurance that the candidate is capable of fulfilling the requirements of the

post. However, breaks for illness and retraining after poor performance reviews can be compensated for by a good service record after returning to work, and doctors in this position may need to choose their jobs carefully to demonstrate their competence and ability.

Overseas trained and refugee doctors

For a large number of overseas trained doctors and refugee doctors, information on the structure of the health service and the alternative options open to doctors may provide a vital first step in working in the UK.[5] The organisation of the NHS will differ significantly from the health service they are used to in their country of origin. Information about the principles underlying UK clinical guidelines and protocols, referral pathways, patient expectations, the career structure for doctors in different parts of the UK, the way in which doctors are paid, and initiatives such as appraisal and revalidation should all be provided, as many of these doctors will find these areas confusing.[6] In addition, these doctors need information that is specific to their situation as international doctors. Such information should cover GMC registration as a doctor in the UK, work permits and the limitations that coming from abroad will have on the options open to them. Qualifications from different parts of the world should be discussed and the role of further training if needed. In particular, doctors from the European Economic Area (EEA) are entitled to enter the UK freely and work here, compared to different regulations applying to doctors coming to the UK from the rest of the world.[7] There are reciprocal agreements in place with some countries (e.g. an agreement exists between the Royal Australian College of General Practitioners and the Royal College of General Practitioners in the UK, that allows mutual recognition of each others' membership examinations).

This group of doctors will require information on how to do the Professional and Linguistic Assessment Board (PLAB) tests,[8] a necessary precursor to working in the UK for many and, for those who first language is not English, the IELTS examination (International English Language Testing System).[9] Being able to access information such as downloadable handbooks or information sheets are often a good place to start,[10–12] although these should also be available in paper format for those doctors coming from parts of the world without readily available internet access. The size and format of the documents should reflect the likely internet connection speed (which can be as low as 28.8 bps dial-up in some parts of the world). Unpaid observation posts or clinical placements may help, *see* Box 3.6.

The Refugee Doctors' Database (further information available from the Refugee Council) contains information derived from refugee doctors who voluntarily participate in the project by sending their details.[13] Collated information is used to facilitate the commissioning of services for this group of doctors, who can then be informed of new services as they are developed.

Box 3.6:   How you might respond to a specific FAQ: I would like to visit the UK
to see what medicine in this country involves prior to obtaining a work permit.
How do I do this?

Many people use an unpaid observation post as a way to see whether they want
to go through the process of getting accredited to work in the UK. Such posts
provide a possible way of obtaining UK references.

   Obtaining such positions depends upon having UK contacts. Family members
or connections from a medical school or hospital in the home country can help
with introductions. It is the personal responsibility of the supervising consultant to be assured that you are a suitable observer.

Underperforming doctors

Increasingly, formal mechanisms are being put in place by trusts and other primary
care organisations to ascertain if doctors are underperforming. Appraisal and revalidation systems are likely to further increase the numbers of doctors requiring
external help or local mentoring or educational input to improve their work.

   Doctors who are categorised as 'underperforming' will need information about
obtaining appropriate support, and help with the effects of difficulties they are
experiencing in relation to their work. You can gain insights into the difficulties
such doctors experience from the published reports of the National Clinical Assessment Service (NCAS), formerly the National Clinical Assessment Authority.[14] They
may need retraining, and the information you supply in conjunction with that of
the trust manager concerned with their case should include contact details of relevant individuals in the local deanery, or the postgraduate tutor in their specialty,
mentoring services and peer support groups. In many cases they will require further
advice and counselling and relevant contact information – advise them to try the
NCAS's toolkit and database of resources.[14]

   Directing these doctors towards locally available training in personal effectiveness,
clinical skills, risk management, and other educational courses may be of help.

How should you make careers information available?

Printed material

Much careers information comes in paper-based form, but there are significant cost
implications involved in posting it out to postgraduate education centres, surgeries,
training schemes, and libraries. Individual doctors most likely to need it (locums, non-
principals, doctors without a fixed NHS base) often miss out unless there is a central
register of names and addresses so that individuals can receive their own copy.
Having sent the information out, updated versions need to be made available on a
regular basis, as careers opportunities and requirements change frequently.

   There are some good books and information guides (*see* references in Chapter 1 and
others[15-17]) to signpost medical students and doctors to.

The internet

A useful way of providing careers information is through the internet, where doctors can access a central website conveniently at work or home, anywhere in the country or abroad. Information can be updated, and the planned availability of NHS net in every health setting makes the internet option feasible. Use of the internet facilitates instant updates and can be easily linked to other sources of information and support both on and away from the web. Ensure that doctors without access to high-speed or reliable internet connections have the option to obtain information by more trad-itional paper-based means. Remember that medical students or doctors in hospital medicine hoping to move into general practice may have limited access to the internet, and alternative means of accessing the information still need to be available.

Trusts and other primary care organisations, deaneries and SHAs do need to put aside funds to cover maintenance costs of the website and ensure it remains up to date at all times.

The *BMJ* boasts a range of careers information for doctors in the UK through its weekly publication of BMJCareers and its associated website.[18]

There is already a great deal of web-based information for those hoping to become doctors, for qualified doctors hoping to pursue a particular specialty, for doctors later in their careers or for doctors moving to the UK from abroad. It is provided by a range of organisations, including the GMC, BMA, Department of Health, Royal Colleges and private companies. The overall quality is high, but, as with all web-based material, check the quality and date of the information provided, before you distribute it to doctors seeking help from you.

The NHS website that provides a range of information on medical careers is at www.nhscareers.nhs.uk/careers/doctors. This site is divided into: working in the NHS, the NHS team – career options, and education and training. It provides information on career options, career path entry requirements, links to relevant organisations and case studies. The information is aimed principally at people considering a career in medicine, but does include some information for qualified doctors too.

The BMA and its associated journal have sites that give extensive information on doctors' careers in the UK. They include survey information and answers to frequently asked questions. Look at www.bmj.com, www.bmjcareers.com, and www.bmj classified.com. They are an excellent place to start a search for careers information.

Doctors will find accounts written by existing doctors of their posts interesting. Some medical schools go further and offer a scheme in which potential or existing students can converse with a qualified doctor (for example, St George's medical school[19]).

For overseas doctors, the University of Manchester provides a number of links to sites that give detailed information about working as a doctor in the UK.[20] The University of Oxford has a database of survey information on this.[21,22] Individual colleges provide information specifically for overseas doctors such as the Royal College of Surgeons.[23]

The GMC offers information on continuing professional development for doc-tors.[24,25]

If you decide to provide careers information via the internet, it should be accessible and easy to navigate. In many instances, simple static HTML pages will convey the information you wish to give effectively, and will work on most browsers. Look at successful sites for inspiration, e.g. www.bmjcareers.com, and focus on local infor-mation that is not available elsewhere on the internet.

For larger careers information sites, the development of dynamic web content allows websites to create information in pages that are tailor-made to the needs of the individual, using one of many commercially available search engines. Accessing this information is easy for the user, and does not require the type of literature search skills that are needed in literature search engines. Dependent upon choices made on earlier pages, doctors can be directed to areas with a clinical or academic emphasis, and traditional or portfolio careers. An example of such a dynamic site is provided by the British Medical Association.[26]

The internet provides an opportunity for doctors who seek careers information to discuss their experiences and learn from each other, through online discussion forums. You may wish to set up such a facility for your local doctors or a group who have characteristics in common. Many people also find the relative anonymity of online discussions less inhibiting than face-to-face discussion. However, such discussions do need to be moderated in order to ensure that the service is used for the purpose for which it was intended, and to provide individuals with links to other sources of support.

Anticipating doctors' information needs

Doctors and medical students consulting you for information about their future careers will not always be aware of what they need to know. You can partly counter this by signposting them to general websites and wide-ranging advice such as that already referred to earlier in this chapter. Your familiarity with and experience of NHS careers should also help you to suggest information that could be useful to them that they have not thought of. A good example might be informing doctors in training of the core competencies that are assessed at selection interviews for training posts. Box 3.7 describes the core competencies assessed at a regional selection process for GP registrars. The accompanying article describes the format of the selection process and approach to scoring.

Box 3.7:   Core competencies assessed at selection of future GP registrars in the West Midlands region[27]

- Communication skills
- Clinical knowledge and expertise
- Enthusiasm
- Punctuality
- Personal organisation and administrative skills
- Professional integrity
- Empathy and sensitivity
- Commitment to general practice
- Takes responsibility
- Seeks help appropriately
- Commitment to learning
- Problem solving
- Teamworking

Similarly, a doctor aspiring to a career move to a manager role, or who has already become a clinical manager and is unaware of the competencies that the job entails if they are to be effective, should benefit from the careers adviser indicating what areas career development should span (*see* Box 3.8).

Box 3.8:   Competencies for medical managers[28]

- Leadership
- Strategic vision
- Personal development skills
- Organisational management skills
- Change and project management skills
- Educational knowledge and skills
- Communicating, influencing, facilitating
- And many more ...

What organisations could help you to provide careers information?

Careers information is probably best delivered centrally by deaneries, or interested SHAs in parallel with Royal Colleges who are well placed to commission follow-on support if doctors need it, and to maintain a service over a long period of time. Trusts and other primary care organisations can provide information about local posts and career options. *See* Chapter 2 for an in-depth review and plan for a comprehensive career management model.

Doctors access careers information in a wide range of ways – from local to web-based resources. However, the most likely method is via personal contacts with colleagues whose opinions they trust. In many cases, these colleagues are not personally experienced in the careers options that interest the doctor concerned, but instead act as an initial source of experience from which the doctor will make decisions about whether they are interested in finding out more and seeking further careers support.

Employing organisations should ensure that a support pathway is available for individual tutors, trainers, supervisors, appraisers etc, to direct the doctor on to where reliable careers information, careers advice or guidance and counselling can be found.

References

1   Chambers R and Mohanna K (2003) Nature of knowledge and skills that might be pertinent to people providing career support to doctors. *BMJ Career Focus.* **326:** 193–4.

2   Department of Health (2004) *Flexible Career Scheme.* www.dh.gov.uk/PolicyAndGuidance/ HumanResourcesAndTraining/MoreStaff/FlexibleCareerScheme/fs/en (accessed 9 August 2005).

3   Lambert T, Davidson JM, Evans J *et al.* (2003) Doctors' reasons for rejecting initial choices of specialties as long-term careers. *Medical Education.* **37:** 312–18.

4   www.bmjcareers.com/advicezone (accessed 9 August 2005).

5   West Midlands Deanery (2004) *International doctors – non-UK graduates.* www.careers. pgmd.man.ac.uk/home/usefulinformation/internationaldoctorsnonukgraduates_ internationaldoctorsnonukgraduatesoverseasinformation.aspx (accessed 9 August 2005).

6   Dosani S and Cross P (2004) *Making it in British Medicine.* Radcliffe Publishing, Oxford.

7   MacDonald R (ed) (2004) *Overseas Doctors: sink or swim?* Career focus information booklet. *BMJcareers.* www.bmjcareers.com (accessed 9 August 2005).

8   General Medical Council (2004) *The Professional and Linguistic Assessments Board (PLAB) Test.* www.gmc-uk.org/register/plab.htm (accessed 9 August 2005).

9   British Council (2004) *IELTS Australia, and University of Cambridge ESOL Examination, International English Language Testing System.* www.ielts.org (accessed 9 August 2005).

10 West Midlands Deanery (2004) *Handbook for Overseas Doctors.* www.pgmd.man.ac.uk/ interdocs/HandbookforOverseasDrs.PDF (accessed 9 August 2005).

11 British Medical Association (2004) *Guide for Doctors New to the UK.* BMA, London.

12 NHS Careers (2003) *NHS International Medical Recruitment: case studies.* NHS Careers, London. www.nhscareers.nhs.uk (accessed 9 August 2005).

13 Refugee Council (2004) *Refugee Doctors' Database.* www.refugeecouncil.org.uk/ downloads/doctor%20database%20leaflet.pdf (accessed 11 October 2005).

14 National Clinical Assessment Authority (2004) *Understanding Performance Difficulties in Doctors.* NCAA, London. www.ncaa.nhs.uk (accessed 9 August 2005).

15 MacDonald R (2003) Where to next? Career focus information guide. *BMJcareers* supplement. www.bmjcareers.com (accessed 9 August 2005).

16 MacDonald R (2003) Pick 'n' mix: career opportunities for GPs. Career focus information guide. *BMJcareers* supplement. www.bmjcareers.com (accessed 9 August 2005).

17 Ciechan J, Girgis S and Smith P (2004) *The Insiders' Guide to Medical Schools.* Blackwell Publishing, London.

18 www.bmjcareers.com (accessed 9 August 2005).

19 www.sgu.edu/EMC/alumniSearch.nsf/findit?OpenForm (accessed 9 August 2005).

20 www.careers.pgmd.man.ac.uk/home/usefulinformation/internationaldoctorsnonuk graduates_internationaldoctorsnonukgraduatesoverseasinformation.aspx (accessed 9 August 2005).

21 www.uhce.ox.ac.uk/ukmcrg (accessed 9 August 2005).

22 www.pubmedcentral.nih.gov/articlerender.fcgi?artid=516656 (accessed 15 August 2005).

23 www.rcseng.ac.uk/career/internationaldoctors/ (accessed 7 October 2005).

24 www.gmc-uk.org/med_ed/cpd/guidance.htm (accessed 9 August 2005).

25 www.gmc-uk.org/revalidation (accessed 9 August 2005).

26 www.bmjcareersadvicezone.synergynewmedia.co.uk (accessed 9 August 2005).

27 Wakefield S (2002) Selecting general practitioner registrars: the West Midlands model. *BMJ Careers.* **6 July:** s3–4.

28 Peskett S and Empey D (2003) A career check for medical managers. *BMJ Careers.* **6 December:** s179–80.

4

What careers advice or guidance should you make available to doctors?

Judi Thorley, Ruth Chambers and Kay Mohanna

Defining the scope of what constitutes careers advice or guidance is crucial. Careers guidance is personal and directive, and provides *advice* within the context of the opportunities that are available. The focus for each individual seeking advice and support will be different. You need to be sure of the limit of your skills, post and responsibility for providing careers advice. You will need to know when to signpost an individual doctor onto other sources of help or information, or refer to someone else. The doctor who has marital or childcare problems, or a drug or alcohol problem may be using difficulties within their career as a way to avoid addressing the real issue. So, you could be faced with someone looking for some help which cannot be offered within a careers advice session, but falls within the scope of career counselling, offered by other trained and competent career counsellors. Box 4.1 summarises the scope of careers advice or guidance for doctors and outlines the type and depth of knowledge and skills you will need.[1]

Box 4.1: Scope of careers advice or guidance[1]

Aspect 1: Guidance about career opportunities
Description: knows how and is able to provide advice and guidance within the context of the opportunities that are available to an individual doctor. (Depth of knowledge and skills range from general awareness of provision of careers advice or guidance to knowing how and being able to give careers advice and guidance appropriate to an individual at any stage of their career for any personal circumstances, with variations of part and full-time working.)

Aspect 2: Setting limits on careers advice or guidance
Description: knows how and is able to contain advice or guidance within limits of the scope of role relating to career guidance. (Depth of knowledge and skills range from general awareness of need to set limits on careers guidance, to knowing how and being able to set limits on the extent of careers advice and guidance however complex or demanding the individual is, and at any stage in their career.)

Aspect 3: Being able to help others derive the information and advice they need to enable them to make career choices

Description: knows how and is able to help others formulate questions to ask and access sources of information and advice to enable them to make informed decisions about career choices. (Depth of knowledge and skills range from general awareness of how to help others formulate questions and access information and advice, to knowing how and being able to help others in that way for a wide range of specialties and personal circumstances.)

Aspect 4: Being able to dovetail provision of careers advice and guidance in own specialty or setting with that from others from other specialties or settings

Description: knows how and is able to link nature of careers advice and guidance provided with that available from others in different specialties and health settings. (Depth of knowledge and skills range from general awareness of linking careers advice and guidance from others to knowing how and being able to link provision of careers advice and guidance with others from wide range of different specialties and health settings in synchronised way covering all stages of the medical career.)

Doctors' experience of receiving careers advice or guidance

It is all too common to find that established doctors have received little in the way of well-informed careers advice and support such as Box 4.2 shows.[2]

Box 4.2:   Comments from doctors about the careers advice they have received

'Never really had any to be honest.'

'I think the bad thing about it is that I haven't had lots of advice at all.'

'As far as careers advice is concerned I've had nothing at all!'

Giving careers advice or guidance is integral to appraisal and supervision

Working within the NHS, doctors and other health professionals are encouraged to develop a 'nurturing' approach to students and junior colleagues. Provision of careers advice is intrinsic within many posts. Organisations expect that more experienced practitioners will support less experienced or novice practitioners to develop, both professionally and personally. To develop this supportive relationship, structures such as personal review, appraisal, reflection and clinical supervision are in place, and practitioners are encouraged to use these. This type of support often takes the form of reflection, encouraging the individual seeking support and advice to reflect back on what they are saying and thinking, to formulate their own pathway forward. But those giving such careers advice or guidance are rarely trained to do so, and their advice may be biased and misleading as a consequence.

Active listening and reflection are key

You may well have been involved in providing some level of careers support in the past and facilitated colleagues' reflection upon their careers, encouraging them to formulate their own way forward, but supported by you. Resisting the temptation to be directive is a highly developed skill. A good careers adviser will learn and practise the skill of active listening, allowing the doctor being guided the time to describe where they are at, and prompting them to find and answer their own questions. A structured reflection model can help you to develop this skill and support the doctor to reach his or her own decisions.

There are many structured reflection models available which provide a framework to support active reflection on either a critical incident or a person's functioning as a whole.[3,4] You need to separate feelings and thoughts from the actual content of a situation or the individual doctor,[3] then understand your potential impact upon the individual doctor for the outcome to be meaningful.

Underperforming doctors

As an appraiser or educator you may not be the best person to advise an underperforming doctor about their career, as your responsibility is to provide a different kind of support or monitoring. *You* may have to advise them to stop practising if you believe patient safety is threatened, or take further action with the authorities if they continue to practise. You may organise for them to be offered more in-depth career counselling where they can consider the circumstances of their underperformance and any mismatch between their personality, beliefs or skills and their career.

What attributes do you need as a careers adviser or guide?

The attributes listed in Box 4.3 describe the qualities that doctors working within primary care in one study have identified as necessary for the doctors providing them with careers advice and support.[2] Being supportive, open, able to ask questions, probe, reflect, challenge, facilitate, guide and encourage are key to your competence and success as a careers adviser.

Box 4.3:   Summary of attributes desired by doctors in a careers adviser or guide[2]

- *Listening skills*: have the ability to actively listen to what is being said, to use vocalisation and silence to encourage the person being listened to, with good non-verbal communication.
- *Experience*: have accumulated knowledge and life experience equipping a person with a range of skills; have experience of being a doctor (in the same setting as the doctor being advised) so as to understand the issues.

- *Credibility*: be capable of being believed, and perceived as trustworthy.
- *Time*: have the time protected to provide careers advice and support.
- *Challenge*: be able to question a statement or fact.
- *Probe*: be able to search for or prompt further information, by thorough inquiry.
- *Honest and trustworthy*: be respected and characterised by sincerity; be reliable, honest and dependable.
- *Knowledge and information*: know sufficient facts about alternative career pathways and have experience.
- *Facilitation*: assist in the progress of career development; encourage thinking and understanding.
- *Empathy*: have the power of understanding and imaginatively entering into another person's feelings.

Doctors' views on careers advisers' attributes

Listening and communication skills

The doctors surveyed in one study of the extent of careers support available emphasised that careers advisers should have good listening skills (*see* Box 4.4). Communication as an aid to understanding the needs and expectations of the individual is a crucial part of the careers advice process. A good interpersonal relationship needs to be established so that careers advice can take place. Other aspects of good communication include having the ability to probe and challenge, pointing out a person's weaknesses and strengths.

Box 4.4:[2]

'They do have to be open, they have to be able to listen.'

'... empathic, a good listener and very non-critical, supporting and positive.'

'Good consultation skills, listening, reflecting and enquiring, clarification etc.'

'You have to get the engagement, the trust, the active listening, ability to reflect, ability to hear what's been said, look at what people are avoiding in conversation, look at when and why they change the subject.'

'You have to feel someone has listened to you and knows what you are like as a person, to then give advice that is valid.'

'They have to be open, they have to be able to listen and have the knowledge to be able to guide.'

'They need to be communicators, listeners ... they would need to be able to seek out a person's weaknesses and strengths.'

Experience

In the main, doctors seem to expect those giving them careers advice to have experience of the NHS, if not to be a doctor themselves, as respondents relate in Box 4.5.[2]

Box 4.5:[2]

'A doctor (providing good careers advice) would understand the problems. People who have been through things already know what the reality is.'

'As a GP I know the stresses they are under, if asked would I feel happy about counselling nurses in their careers the answer would be no because I couldn't relate to their experiences and background.'

'Someone who has been there and done it, experienced the options, preferably found positive ways through it.'

'Somebody who has experience and knowledge.'

Credibility

Linked to experience is the credibility arising from the careers adviser also having had a health service career or being senior or having achieved in their field (*see* Box 4.6).

Box 4.6:[2]

'I think credibility is important ... sometimes it's about what you've done outside of that role, they know what you're like when you're with them at a meeting or speak to them on the phone.'

'I think if somebody has got medical experience themselves who is still working, they obviously can relate to your problems and frustrations and can understand why and what you want to do.'

Protecting time

You can only provide careers advice or guidance if you have the dedicated time to do it – as in Box 4.7.

Box 4.7:[2]

'Also the concept of protected time. It is important from a professional point of view and to enable you to do your job properly.'

'There should be protected time for it. It should be built into the SHO rotation for instance. One afternoon or something.'

'Time is an expensive commodity particularly if it is a doctor providing the careers advice.'

'Whatever you do in medicine it is incredibly hectic. We don't make time to take our own careers on board. We don't value careers advice.'

'... if you want to do it then you make the time. Time of course is the big issue. That is the nice thing about appraisals, you actually set aside the time, you are actually paid to do it, you make the time.'

'Once somebody has said this has got to happen then the time is made. I think time is less of an issue than saying "Yes, this is important, we must make time for it." '

'People often put up barriers, one barrier is the threat, and the second barrier is a perceived weakness that you need help, but the most common barriers are time and money. So we need protected time to do these things.'

Challenging

One of the most important facets of giving careers advice or guidance to a doctor, or anyone else, is to challenge their beliefs or current practice. This should open up new thinking and enable them to explore new possibilities – as in Box 4.8.

Box 4.8:[2]

'Also challenging because we often don't get challenged ... There is nothing wrong with feeling that, but let us look at why you have those feelings and reflect on the reasons.'

'Sometimes people want to change their job because of things to do with the GP partnership – often they just want to talk that through with somebody – the partnership they have is fine, is it just they need to work around it?'

'To tease out and explore the things that people touched on and try to decide whether those were important things or throwaway remarks. Getting down to the nitty-gritty with people, asking for examples.'

'Someone who doesn't go along with everything you say but needs to see where you are coming from. For example, you say you want to become this, is it because you want to become that or is it a dream ... It's about challenging.'

'Where do you want to be in five years time? And knowing you want to be there, how are you going to get there?'

Probing

Linked to challenge is probing. A good careers adviser will adopt a probing approach, to encourage the doctor who is consulting them to explore areas of their thinking or aspirations in depth – as in Box 4.9.

Box 4.9:[2]

'She is a very good listener and very good at asking open-ended questions, which make you think.'

'Someone who doesn't go along with everything that you say. For example, when you say you want to become X, well is it because you want that or is it because you are just so sick and tired of where you are now?'

'I think it would make people reflect more on the career options. I think it is a very good way to make you think about ways of improving things.'

'Good consultation skills, listening, reflecting, and enquiring, clarification and stuff like that. It's helping to form the discussion in a way that says, let's recap and what are the outcomes from this and where do we go from here?'

'I see it as just a time, space and an opportunity for somebody to explore issues with someone else and find out more about things for themselves.'

Honesty and trust

You can only expect people to trust you as a careers adviser if you are honest with them. That may include describing any conflicts of interest you have got, such as the hope that you will be able to retain them in their current job. The quotes in Box 4.10 shows how important the qualities of honesty and trust are.

Box 4.10:[2]

'Just that there have been people I knew and trusted and who I thought were quite good at what they were doing, I valued their opinions.'

'He is very empathic, a good listener and very non-critical, supporting and positive.'

'You need to be able to trust them and have confidence in them. Like an appraiser, you need to feel comfortable with them. Obviously somebody who has experience and knowledge, it is important that they treat you as an equal.'

'It has got to be somebody who can be trusted by their colleagues, otherwise they will not speak their minds and they can end up in unhappy jobs – jobs they were never really meant to be going into.'

'I like transparency and honesty. I would rather have honesty even if it makes me feel a little upset.'

'Respect is very important. You don't always have to get on with people but as long as you have that in a working relationship.'

Knowledge and information

You will need to have a background knowledge about different career options in medicine, length of training, how to train, what qualifications you need etc – or know where to get that reliable information from, or signpost them to – as in Box 4.11.

Box 4.11:[2]

'It would have to be someone who is very well informed with knowledge of the options available.'

'... tell them where they need to go for support. There are some people who might need advice and there are others who might just need information.'

'They would need to have quite a clear understanding about the different attributes of a personality that make people better fit for one type of work than another ... they would need to know the types of tools available to help people work through what their own particular personality types are.'

'It may not be handing everything on a plate, but saying – I know where the resources are that you need or I know where the information is ... I think you have got to have a certain basic minimum knowledge.'

'They have to have good communication skills. They have got to understand all the different branches of medicine and what the careers require and what the development pathways are.'

Facilitation

If you are not to be directive, you need skills in facilitation to enable others to explore and make career choices – *see* what respondents want in Box 4.12.

Box 4.12:[2]

'Careers advice is about support, it is guidance and it is that encouragement word again. I think the encouragement is really important because, you are the only one that can do it at the end of the day.'

'Good consultation skills, listening, reflecting and enquiring, clarification and stuff like that, it's just guiding the interview if you like, guiding the discussion, rather than guiding the outcome.'

'Allowing people space to expand and asking specific questions.'

'As well as identifying personality traits it is about identifying drives and ambitions and what somebody wants to achieve, find out what they want to do and what they feel is stopping them doing it.'

'... as an appraiser I see myself as a sort of mirror where you reflect things back onto the appraisee to help them determine where they are at the moment, what they hope to do and what tools they need to do that.'

Empathy

Being a careers adviser or guide is not just about your knowledge and skills and the back up information about career options. It is about having the right attitude and showing empathy too (*see* Box 4.13).

Box 4.13:[2]

'The person needs to be empathetic and probably needs to be quite charming in order to work with doctors.'

'It's about being empathic, supportive. Someone who doesn't go along with everything you say but needs to see where you are coming from.'

'They obviously can relate to your problems and frustrations and can understand why and what you want to do, [they are] approachable, somebody that you feel comfortable talking to.'

'If medical students get really worried I might say to them "look if you don't pass the first time don't worry because I failed everything and still got here in the end", I sometimes use that example.'

'I guess we ought to look at the attitudes of careers advisers as well. It has to be non-judgemental and supportive. Also, to recognise that people aren't always going to make the best fit career choice because there are other demands in their lives.'

Being effective as a careers adviser or guide

For a careers advice session to be effective the doctor acting as careers adviser will need many, if not all, of the attributes described in Boxes 4.3 to 4.13. Having a 'tool box' which is stocked with this range of skills will take time to develop. Doctors who are in the position of careers adviser need to be familiar with their personal style and preferred approach. It may be useful if they have completed a personality type indicator test themselves (*see* page 90). That should give them more insight into their interactions with the doctors they are advising, so that their sessions are effective with a range of doctors with varied personalities and different circumstances. For example if as an adviser your personal style is to be extrovert in your thinking, then you may tend to become irritated with the doctor who prefers not to share information during a session. Your approach in this situation might be to give them 'homework' so that they can concentrate on the issues when alone, which they may then feel more able to share at your next meeting.

You will be taking the careers discussion further in order to help the individual doctor to prioritise their needs, career goals and aspirations – the key approach to providing effective careers advice and support. Developing the ability to challenge others to enable them to understand the unconscious reasons for their decision making is crucial to achieve their expectations and goals set at your initial meeting. Engaging in a two-way process of communication is essential to creating a positive experience for other doctors within the context of careers advice.

Careers advisers will come to the role with a range of experience and levels of expertise. What they all share is the need to develop that expertise and hone their skills in the important area of interpersonal communication. Communication skills from consulting with patients are transferable to a greater extent, and are a good basis for developing the right attributes as a careers guide. Those interested in developing active listening skills might choose to follow the exercises suggested in a self-assessment and development resource in communication skills, published by the Royal College of General Practitioners,[5] or to participate in a communications skills training course.

You can think more about what it means to be competent and how to demonstrate that you are competent to provide careers information and advice in Chapter 9.

Ground rules and careers advice 'contract'

Agreeing ground rules and setting a date for review is crucial for the careers advice process to be beneficial. Consider:

- agreeing what does and does not constitute careers advice or guidance
- agreeing the purpose of careers advice session(s). Discuss their expectations in full
- deciding the duration of session; and if you meet again, the frequency and venue
- agreeing on honest and open discussion, and boundaries of confidentiality
- limiting interruptions – in particular mobile phones
- how to make appropriate careers information available
- agreeing that either party can withdraw from the careers advice session(s) without giving reasons.

References

1 Chambers R and Mohanna K (2003) Nature of knowledge and skills that might be pertinent to people providing career support to doctors. *BMJ Career Focus.* **326:** 193–4s.

2 Thornett A, Thorley J and Chambers R (2005) *Providing Careers Support for Rural General Practitioners – the competencies of careers advisors* (in press).

3 Egan G (1990) *The Skilled Helper* (6e). Brooks Cole Publishing Co, New York.

4 Chambers R (ed) (2005) *Career Planning for Everyone in the NHS. The toolkit.* Radcliffe Publishing, Oxford.

5 Mohanna K (2005) *Self-assessment Workbook for Appraisers.* Royal College of General Practitioners, London.

5

Training and developing careers advisers

Andrew Thornett and Ruth Chambers

Developing competency: novice to expert

Competence is about being 'able to perform the tasks and roles required to the expected standard'.[1] So, knowledge and skill are components of competence. Capability is a term that describes 'what a person can think or do'. Whether or not a person's capability makes them competent in a particular job such as being a careers adviser depends on them being able to meet the requirements of that job.[2] Capability implies that individuals can develop sustainable abilities that allow them to adapt to a changing environment and react appropriately to unfamiliar situations.

The standard expected to be able to judge someone as 'competent' will vary with their experience and level of responsibility, and take into account the need to keep up to date with changes in practice. Different people will have varied expectations of what counts as competence – managers, staff, individuals, patients, clients, etc.

There can be a gap between competence – what a person can do – and performance – what a person actually does. This gap can be caused by a range of factors – personal matters such as an individual's attitude or personality or mood, environmental factors such as workload, time pressures or working conditions, or situational factors such as a lack of resources or support.

In the Benner hierarchy competence can be graded in six stages ranging from *irrelevant* to *novice* to *expert*:[3,4]

1 *irrelevant to post*
2 *novice*: beginners have no experience of the situations in which they are expected to perform
3 *advanced beginner*: the advanced beginner can demonstrate marginally acceptable performance
4 *competent*: competence is being able to perform the tasks and roles required to the expected standard (e.g. of providing careers information, advice or guidance as described in Chapters 3 and 4)
5 *proficient*: the proficient person learns from experience what typical events to expect in a given situation and how plans need to be modified in response to these events
6 *expert*: the expert has an enormous background of experience, an intuitive grasp of each situation and zeroes in on the problem without wasteful consideration of a

large range of unfruitful, alternative diagnoses and solutions. An expert interprets and synthesises information, and can handle a wide range of problems in different contexts.

As you consolidate your knowledge and skills and positive attitude as a careers adviser and gain experience you should move from:

*   novice or advanced beginner towards competent
*   competent towards proficient
*   proficient towards expert.

Training of careers support personnel

The training you require to provide careers support depends upon whether you provide careers information, advice or counselling, and the particular group of doctors for which you provide support. Your professional background and experience will affect your training needs too.

The deaneries, SHAs, trusts and other primary care organisations that employ careers support personnel should ensure that their knowledge and skills remain up to date and relevant to doctors seeking their advice.

Much of the training will be 'on the job' and via learning activities described in your PDP. You might start by recognising the knowledge and skills you already possess that are relevant to providing careers information and advice or guidance, and then defining what else is needed according to the competencies you need for the advisory role (*see* page 24). There are no specific careers guidance qualifications for providing careers advice to doctors. National careers guidance qualifications awarded by the Institute of Career Guidance take a year full-time or two years of part-time study. They prepare the career guidance specialist for the general career guidance sector, including Connexions/careers services in England and other careers services within further and higher education institutes across the UK, providing information, advice and guidance for adults etc.

Training for careers advisers should aim to achieve the learning outcomes in Box 5.1. An example programme for an initial training workshop is given in Appendix 3. These learning outcomes seek to enable you, as a careers adviser of doctors, to provide tailored advice or guidance that facilitates a doctor's development as an individual. Your training needs to help you to assist doctors in making decisions about their careers, and enable you to develop in them the knowledge and skills they require to continue developing their careers, even when you are not present. You might start with an initial workshop from which you draw up a PDP working with a colleague or deanery-based careers lead to attain the learning outcomes of Box 5.1 over time.

Box 5.1:   The learning outcomes of a training programme for careers advisers

*   Be able to deliver impartial advice or guidance on career choices.
*   Be able to provide informed guidance on an individual's suitability for specific medical careers.
*   Understand the importance of critical junctures within the training and qualifications structure.
*   Be able to provide both clinically related careers advice or guidance and human resource guidance (e.g. for CV, interview skills) at local level.

- Understand the information, advice and guidance needs of doctors at all stages of their careers.
- Understand the information, advice and guidance requirements of doctors with specific career needs.
- Have a flexible ethos, to enable doctors to recognise the uncertain nature of their future career in a continually changing NHS.

The range of depth of knowledge and skills you will need is summarised in Box 5.2. These are derived from the NHS Knowledge and Skills Framework (KSF) expected of anyone working in the NHS.[5] These tally well with the qualities and attributes that doctors want in a careers adviser (*see* Box 4.3) and in addition offer the wider perspective – such as skills in treating people equally, valuing diversity, promoting a high standard of performance at work, and contributing to good local careers information and advice services.

An advantage of basing the knowledge and skills of a careers adviser on this framework is that if the careers adviser is also employed as an appraiser or mentor, job descriptions and competencies for all roles can also be based on the KSF. This makes it easy to see which knowledge and skills are transferable between the various roles, and for which extra training and development or prior experience is needed. Other parallel work has been done to define job descriptions for appraisers and mentors of doctors based on the KSF.[6–9]

For each of these knowledge and skills summarised in Box 5.2, you can progress from general awareness that these should be part of a good careers adviser's qualities (that is the *novice* or *advanced beginner* of the Benner hierarchy given on pages 45–6) to being *competent*, *proficient* and eventually *expert* when you are able to provide careers advice or guidance to doctors and medical students in complicated situations, such as those experiencing career crises (*see* page 59) or who are underperforming or referred to you because of particular concerns.

Box 5.2: Brief descriptions of the six core dimensions of the knowledge and skills as relevant to a provider of careers information, advice or guidance to medical students or doctors[5]

1 *Communication*: consistently practise good communication skills.
2 *Personal and people development*: develop own skills and knowledge and provide information and advice to others to help their development.
3 *Health, safety and security*: assist in maintaining others' health, safety and security.
4 *Service development*: contribute to the improvement of NHS services (through effective careers information/advice).
5 *Quality improvement*: demonstrate personal commitment to quality improvement, offering others advice and support.
6 *Equality and diversity*: act in ways that support equality and value diversity.

Providing careers information

If you provide careers information, then your training should be directed at obtaining the knowledge about where information can be found on the range of careers options available to doctors working in primary or secondary care. This should include relevant non-health options as well.

It should concentrate a general awareness of the breadth of options available, with a particular emphasis upon information on local options. In addition, you should have detailed knowledge of sources of information for all specialties, parallel careers, and allied non-health posts. Such training may be provided by formal courses completed prior to starting to provide careers information, and by follow-up training at regular points thereafter so that providers can remain up to date. Alternatively, you could compile a portfolio by independent study. The range and breadth of options, legal and training framework change regularly, and consequently you will need protected time to continue to remain up to date on an ongoing basis.

The knowledge base you develop should include familiarity with the qualifications, training and experience needed to undertake various career options, and the number and type of posts available at all levels, so that doctors who seek information from you are able to make sensible decisions about risk. For many positions in medicine, legislation limits access or plays an important part in determining the nature and content of the job. You need to be aware of current regulations relating to doctors in training and their gaining of qualifications. The extent to which you require such detailed knowledge depends upon the location in which you work, and where those seeking advice from you live and work. In some areas, a detailed knowledge of regulations for professionals who have trained overseas, taken a prolonged career break, have unusual career routes, or want to (re-)enter a particular specialty will be important, while in others being able to direct the professional interested in this information to someone with more information on the issue will be adequate. Access to well-developed, up-to-date websites of information will be vital.

Many students and doctors will value hearing personal experiences of different careers. So be aware of local personnel who are willing to provide such a personal perspective, and be able to provide contact information for them.

Providing careers advice or guidance

As a result of the *Modernising Medical Careers* initiative,[10] trained providers of careers advice and counselling should now be available in all areas of the UK, and all employing organisations in the NHS need to consider how they are going to ensure that their career advisers and counsellors are adequately trained.

Few of those providing careers advice are professionals who will solely or largely provide careers support as their main occupation. For most, it forms part of a much wider range of roles. The diversity of roles undertaken by these professionals has led to inadequate training in providing careers support in the past, and this needs to be remedied. All educational supervisors and clinical tutors should be trained to a minimum level of competence in careers advice and guidance (*see* page 35). Others (such as CPD tutors, course organisers, university staff, deanery staff, mentors, health librarians, trust staff, appraisers, College representatives) should be aware of good practice in the giving of careers information, advice and guidance and careers counselling, and be able to signpost doctors to relevant sources of help.

Training needs to cover the interpersonal skills required to interact with medical professionals in a way that enables successful careers development. Such skills include an ability to relate to the individual doctor's personal and professional situation, and to express empathy and demonstrate understanding – as described in Chapter 4.

For many doctors, career development is a highly stressful undertaking and they need someone who can help them to express their concerns and desires in a manner that leads to identified solutions and realistic career plans. In some situations, the skills required include the ability to use appropriate tools, but often the most important attributes you need as an adviser are the ability to empathise, clarify and restructure thoughts, and to put the doctor at ease when they talk to you. You need to be able to help other doctors to prioritise their needs and wants, and to obtain a clearer indication of where they want to go and how they intend to get there. Consequently, your skills should include a practical ability to see through the maze of information presented in order to determine which aspects of the professional's life are most important for his or her careers decision. Then it is important to be able to present this back in a way which enables the individual to move forward effectively. In many cases, doctors will have worked out to some extent where they want to go, and will only require generic advice. However, for others, more in-depth career counselling is required, and for these individuals the interpersonal skills of the careers support person become particularly important. The training you undertake should enable you to define the limits of careers advice or guidance, and be able to refer needy doctors on to others trained in careers counselling.

In a recent project in the West Midlands, careers advice delivered by HR professionals in addition to medical advisers was greatly valued by the doctors involved.[11] Two types of careers advice were required: advice on career paths and advice on securing a particular post. From this study, it is clear that doctors value information, but they are also keen to receive practical training in how to achieve their goals. Your advice should cover these areas, and also assist doctors in determining whether the practical realities of pursuing particular avenues mitigate against their pursuing those opportunities.

As a careers adviser, it is your responsibility to help trainees who are not suited to a career specialty, or do not have the aptitude for a chosen career path, to gain insight into the mismatch between their career aspirations and reality. Here you may need to arrange career counselling, or be able to employ and interpret personality profile testing to increase a doctor's insight into their own strengths and preferences in conjunction with feedback from the person administering the tests (e.g. Sci45 Specialty Choice Inventory – *see* page 90).[12]

Providing career counselling

The training and development of career counsellors is outside the scope of this book. They should be trained to enable medical students and doctors to come to informed and rational decisions about where to go next. They should be capable of enabling such doctors to reflect on and appreciate their own strengths and weaknesses, and other areas listed in Box 5.3. In many areas, counsellors themselves receive individualised support and mentoring that enables them to reflect upon their own practice in a safe environment, with an emphasis upon formative development.

Box 5.3:   Particular roles of careers counsellors for medical students and doctors

- Remedial action for underperformance
- Generic career counselling as option- not specialty-specific
- Sources of appropriate support
- Facilitation of individual doctors/dentists at times of 'crisis'
- Personality profiling: for doctors with attitudinal and interpersonal problems
- A service that can 'match' a person with a career specialism or mode of working; helping them face up to their lack of suitability for a particular specialism
- Ability to provide help and support for hard truths emanating from career counselling – coming to terms with limited career choices or unwanted insights

---

Probably the most important difference between career counselling and careers advice is that the latter enables doctors to take an active part in planning their own career pathways via access to careers information (paper and electronic), career management workshops, software to help with decision support in careers, and careers advisory services. The former aims to build insights into personal attributes and blocks to development, to allow a person to move forward.

Summary

Deaneries and trusts as employing organisations should enable and ensure that all staff in educationally supportive posts for doctors are competent at providing careers advice. All those providing careers support should be well trained and supported themselves – with access to help and advice in their roles.

As a careers support professional, it is your responsibility to ensure that your knowledge is up to date, and your skills reflect your role as a careers information provider, or adviser. However, you cannot achieve the skills or knowledge required without support from other people in your organisation and without peer support from other careers support professionals. Seek out such support and maintain an active learning programme for yourself, that allows you to continue to deliver high-quality care for doctors who consult you about their careers. Turn to Chapter 8 to consider the various knowledge and skills you will require in more specific detail, and some tools you could use to provide careers advice.

References

1   Eraut M and du Boulay B (2000) *Developing the Attributes of Medical Professional Judgement and Competence.* University of Sussex, Sussex. www.informatics.sussex.ac.uk/users/bend/doh (accessed 9 August 2005).

2   Fraser SW and Greenhalgh T (2001) Coping with complexity: educating for capability. *BMJ.* **323**: 799–802.

3   Benner P (1984) *Novice to Expert.* Addison Wesley, London.

4   Storey L, Howard J and Gillies A (2002) *Competency in Healthcare. A practical guide to competency frameworks.* Radcliffe Medical Press, Oxford.

5   Department of Health (2004) *The NHS Knowledge and Skills Framework (NHS KSF) and the Development Review Process.* Department of Health, London.

6   Chambers R, Tavabie A, Mohanna K and Wakley G (2004) *The Good Appraisal Toolkit for Primary Care.* Radcliffe Publishing, Oxford.

7   Bayley H, Chambers R and Donovan C (2004) *The Good Mentoring Toolkit for Healthcare.* Radcliffe Publishing, Oxford.

8   Chambers R, See S, Tavabie A and Hughes S (2004) Composing a competency-based job description for general practice appraisers using the NHS Knowledge and Skills Framework. *Education for Primary Care.* **15**: 15–29.

9   Chambers R, Tavabie A, See S and Hughes S (2004) Template for a competency-based job description for mentors of GPs using the NHS Knowledge and Skills Framework. *Education for Primary Care.* **15**: 220–30.

10   Department of Health (2004) *Modernising Medical Careers. The next steps.* Department of Health, London.

11   Bullock A and Field S (2004) *Careers Advice for Junior Doctors. Final report.* University of Birmingham, Birmingham.

12   Gale R and Grant J (2002) Sci45: the development of a specialty choice inventory. *Medical Education.* **36**: 659–66.

6

Career self-management: career planning for doctors

Ruth Chambers and Kay Mohanna

We have included a career planning approach in this book to enable doctors and medical students to manage their careers. So we have personalised the content of the chapter so you and others can work through it as an exercise to be sure that you or they are on the right career track. It may be that you as a doctor providing careers information, advice or guidance, might benefit from taking the opportunity to reflect on and plan your career too. Or you might want to enable someone you are advising to reflect on and plan their career – using one or more of the tools in this chapter.

Our tips for any doctor managing their career are:[1,2]

- consider what you want or need from your career and what you can offer in return
- recognise your transferable skills and the competencies you have already developed over time
- develop one or more career goals
- be flexible about change so that you can take advantage of opportunities as they crop up
- promote an accurate profile of yourself: maximise your strengths, acknowledge your weaknesses or inexperience and what you are doing to address these
- understand the value of your contribution to others and their work programmes in various health settings or organisations
- plan for your future – never stop – even if it is to get ready for a fulfilling retirement.

Career analysis for doctors[3]

The following section describes how any doctor might analyse their situation and work along their own career planning pathway to take them from where they are now to where they want to get to, or at least another acceptable stage in a progressive career path. Box 6.1 summarises the main stages. Encourage any doctor to undertake this analysis of their career, by themselves or working through it with a mentor, tutor or trusted colleague. The more they do for themselves, the less input you should need to make as a careers adviser.

Box 6.1:　Stages in career planning

1　Who are you and where are you now?
2　What changes do you want to make?
3　How are you going to get there?
4　What will you do if you don't get what you want or hope for?

The career compass

Who are you and where are you now?

Looking inwards

Consider:

you:

- what are your strengths and weaknesses in your various roles or posts?
- do you understand your own personality: have you undertaken a personality profile test? Do the insights about your personality affect your career choice?
- what transferable skills do you have that might fit you for a different kind of career?
- how does your current work and life measure up to your inner values?
- what kind of roles and responsibilities do you prefer? Do you enjoy leading or following? Do you like to manage or be managed?
- what fears do you have that you need to overcome?
- what qualities do you have that you need to exploit or harness?

your current job:

- do the features of your job fit with your personal style?
- how satisfied are you with your job – working hours, responsibility, location, patient contact, workload, income, challenge, opportunities for change or development, extent of socialising, your skills, on-call commitment, support from colleagues, variety?
- how satisfied are you with your career in general?
- what aspects of work do you value?
- are there inner barriers that hinder your career advancement in your current job (e.g. self-doubt, low self-esteem)?
- do you act the part in your post, even if you do not feel confident?
- do you exceed your job description? You can impress others with your initiative and capability
- do you set yourself new targets within your job to keep your interest alive and provide new challenges?
- do you nurture your relationships with other colleagues? You never know when you may need their support or help.

Looking outwards

Consider:

- what opportunities are there for promotion or other roles or extending your skills, in your current job?
- what opportunities might there be for developing new skills or enhancing current skills in your present job?
- what other jobs are on offer elsewhere for which you might apply?
- what other role(s) and responsibilities do you see yourself taking on?
- have you got enough support from others at work?
- what qualities and skills do others perceive that you have?
- is your potential recognised or realised in your current post?

Looking sideways

Consider:

- how do your current workload and conditions impact on your family and other aspects of your non-working life?
- how satisfied are you with your lifestyle and time spent outside work – sport, relaxation, hobbies, travel?
- how much quality time do you have for friends and family?
- what is the balance like between your current work and other aspects of your life?
- do you have a mentor? A role model or influential colleague might well give your career a boost.

Box 6.2:   What makes you think about leaving?[4]

- What do you dislike about your current job?
- Is it boredom, stress, work overload, relationships, the environment?
- How are these problems affecting you, specifically?
- What would you like less of in your job?
- What would you like more of?
- Have you been here before? Is the problem part of a pattern in your career?
- What will you be looking for in your next job or way of life if you leave?

What changes do you want to make?

Consider:

- to what extent are you content to remain in the same job, practice or NHS trust?
- what makes you think about leaving your current job? *See* Box 6.2 for reasons that may be underlying your wish to quit
- to what extent will your current role satisfy you in one/three years' time – *see* Box 6.3?
- what is it that you most want to achieve? What are your career goals?
- do your career goals conflict with other types of success or fulfilment that you are seeking in other areas of your life (for instance, financial goals, social goals, leisure goals, personal goals in relation to your family)?

- what will be your strengths and skills and achievements by certain time milestones?
- how will you acquire those skills and experience in the meantime to develop your full potential? Skills developed outside work may be just as important as those developed as part of your job
- what resources do you have to help you achieve your career goals?
- applying for promotion to show others that you are motivated to progress your career.

Where do you want to be in ONE year's time?

Write down your goals after reading through the career challenge in Box 6.3.

Box 6.3:   Take a career challenge in formulating your goals

What role do you see yourself doing in three, five, fifteen years' time? Think widely: academic career, research interest or audit, opportunities for teaching, location, preferences or hobbies, access to relatives, alternative and parallel clinical or management work, availability of cover by colleagues, supportive colleagues, sponsors and friends. Do you know of someone whose career pathway or roles you would like to emulate?

Looking inwards:

-
-
-

Looking outwards:

-
-
-

Looking sideways:

-
-
-

Where do you want to be in THREE years' time?
Write down your goals:

Looking inwards:

•

•

•

Looking outwards:

•

•

•

Looking sideways:

•

•

•

How are you going to get there?

Work out the series of steps you will need to take over the next 12 months to achieve your one-year goals; and longer-term action for your three-year or even five- or fifteen-year goals. Think how to make things happen. To whom can you talk to get more information or advice? Who can you visit to see if their type of work appeals to you? Who can give you well-informed careers guidance or career counselling? How can you gain the preliminary achievements and experience that you need?

Getting ready to make a change

What do you need to do first?

- further reflection and review of how satisfied you are with your career, your job, your life in general – as in the section on 'Who are you and where are you now'
- discuss your satisfaction and options with others close to you – at home, your family and friends, work colleagues, trusted advisers and confidantes
- find out more information and facts about other careers or new skills
- ask someone for advice about opportunities in their field and what their jobs entail

- seek further careers information, careers advice or guidance
- make a list of your options and reflect (with someone whose opinion you value) on their relative advantages.

Are you ready to change?

- How positive are you about going ahead and making changes?
- Does what you are proposing fit with your ethics, values and boundaries?
- What is it that has limited you from making changes in the past? Have you overcome those constraints or barriers now?
- Are you clear about what interests and motivates you to work effectively?

So what will you do?

Make your plans happen with timetabled action. Think of:

- setting goals
- what new insights, knowledge, skills and attitudes you need to develop
- using your skills and experience
- your timetable
- how you will proceed
- support and resources you will need to make your plans come to fruition
- overcoming limiting factors: what risks you need to manage
- situations you may wish to influence: to prevent or provoke events or activities.

What will you do if you don't get what you want or hope for?

Write down your contingency plans

For instance:

- how could you change your current job so that you have more job satisfaction?
- re-evaluate your options. What is your 'second choice' alternative career path or career development?
- re-assess your previous goals and objectives
- what other skills might you develop within medicine or in your leisure time?
- could you get more balance into your life by building in more self-development time?
- think again if anyone else might help you through all your networks and contacts.
- can you fit two different jobs into your life, working part-time on each?
- think again about what you really want out of life
- counter any self-defeating beliefs that you have uncovered in undertaking the review of your career
- adopt some better personal stress management in all sections of your life and work
- build up your support mechanisms: at work, with friends, with family and your partner at home.

Work/life balance

Pursuing a fulfilling career should be about working smarter rather than working harder. The work/life balance is now as important to some individuals as any financial rewards. Working longer hours will not necessarily help you to work more effectively. Many people experience a tension between work and home demands, and it is difficult to juggle home and work priorities and set time aside to keep fit and relax. But you must try to achieve a good balance to give you an intellectual edge and help you to maintain your sense of perspective. It requires self-discipline to set personal boundaries, self-confidence to view your time as equally important to that of other people and energy to redesign your daily habits. Career health is dependent on your physical and mental wellbeing and retaining a sense of proportion in terms of what is really important in life. Your career is just one element of your life, so do get it in perspective as for the doctor cited in Box 6.4.

Box 6.4

'If I had worked full-time I never would have seen my husband and childcare was impossible where we lived. Now I could do full-time I don't want to – too old!!'[5]

There are no hard and fast rules about how much time you should spend on work-related activities compared to the rest of your life. Sensible advice is to divide your day as:[6]

- 45–55% on personal needs (including sleeping, chores, basic care)
- 25–30% on work
- 20–25% on leisure.

Only you and your partner at home know if you are getting the balance right. And if you have not got a 'partner at home' to discuss the balance with, maybe it's time you reduced your wholesale commitment to work and socialised more in order to make new friends. If you increase the proportion of work, it is the leisure component that is reduced proportionately.

The impact of your career on those at home

Do not forget the impact of your career choice upon your partner and family at home – if that is relevant to your own circumstances. Your family may not be tolerant of you prioritising your career, or studying for further qualifications or making a house move to take up a different post as for the doctor in Box 6.5.

Box 6.5

'My social circumstances – mother of two small children, working part-time – influence my career decisions far more than availability or otherwise of careers information.'[2]

Factors to consider in choosing a career specialty or interest

When you review your current job or weigh up the potential for a career path or move, consider the match between you and the job as to whether:

- you have the sort of personality that fits with the requirements of the job
- you have the appropriate skills, training and experience
- you have sufficient job satisfaction and interest in your work
- you are sufficiently motivated to work effectively
- the job fits with your ethics, inner values and boundaries
- the job provides the balance you want between work and your off-duty life.

How will you know if you have achieved your career goals if you do not have a vision for the future? Identify what you are aiming for and the nature of the milestones that will describe how you are going to get there. This does not mean that you cannot change your career plan if your circumstances should change; it is essential to your success to be flexible.

Two of the most common reasons given for changing careers in one study were the 'hours of work' and 'working conditions'.[7]

Career crises[8]

A career crisis could be anything that abruptly alters the way you think about your career path. The factors that might temporarily or permanently derail your career can be divided into internal and external factors, and some are listed in Box 6.6. One example might be a doctor developing a physical or mental impairment that interferes with their work sufficiently for it to be difficult for them to continue in their post, or even put patient safety at risk. In that case they will have no choice but to stop work and revise their role and responsibilities within their specialty area or change career to another clinical or non-clinical position.

Box 6.6: Examples of factors that may affect the smooth flow of your career pathway

Internal factors

- Illness, e.g. short-term such as fractured limb; long-term such as depression or chronic condition
- Burnout
- Job dissatisfaction
- Change of priorities, including positive changes
- Pregnancy
- Mismatch with intended career – personality, skills
- As a junior doctor – is medicine for me?
- Sudden deterioration of chronic illness – not allowed to drive

External factors

- Lack of career progression, lack of jobs
- Dealing with complaints that could potentially terminate career

- Immigration rules
- Trust reconfiguration/enforced redundancy
- Discrimination (age, gender, race, disability, pregnancy)
- 'The establishment' – 'old boy network'
- Family's competing needs – housing, education, income, family illness
- Differing career paths of partner (geographic/time)
- Low income as a rural GP with few holidays
- Suspension and investigation by police after death of a patient
- Being suddenly made redundant
- GP partner 'fiddling the books'
- Complete change of weekly timetable by trust
- Unable to get a job after passing PLAB exams
- Personal circumstances change, e.g. divorce, bereavement

Career anchors

Consider what motivates you

People are motivated by different things. Money, fame, power are all key motivators. Pride, lust, anger, gluttony, envy, sloth and covetousness are all listed as prime motivators – hopefully not all of these are relevant to any great extent for you working in the NHS! Some of the best motivators for fulfilling your needs are:

- interesting and/or useful work
- a sense of achievement
- responsibility
- opportunities for career progression or professional development
- gaining new skills or competencies
- a sense of belonging to a directorate or practice team or the NHS in general.

A survey of doctors and medical students found that the same four features of work were most important to the various groups of the 1740 respondents:[9]

- balance between work and home (71% rated this extremely important)
- job satisfaction (66% rated this as extremely important)
- working in a friendly atmosphere (62% rated this extremely important)
- doing a worthwhile job (57% rated this as extremely important).

Opportunities for promotion and good financial rewards were the two features that fewest respondents rated as extremely important to them. Two-thirds of female respondents rated opportunities for flexible working as very or extremely important to them, compared to one-third of male respondents.

Maslow's hierarchy of a person's needs describes how self-esteem and fulfilment are not possible if the basic structure and safety components of their life are insecure.[10] Fulfilment and personal growth are only likely to occur if the basics of an individual's life are in place. Self-esteem, status and recognition from others are only possible if they are built upon a good social base that includes love, friendship, belonging to groups (work, home, leisure, professional), and social activities. Fulfilment, maturity and wisdom are only possible where all the other conditions encourage growth, personal development and accomplishment. If a doctor is contemplating a career change or expansion of their career that will require new skills, knowledge and experiences, they might be better waiting until their personal life is reasonably settled and they feel secure, before making major alterations or moving on.

Consider what is important to you as a professional. The ability to critically appraise your own strengths and weaknesses, aptitudes and values as a person and as a healthcare professional is vital if you are to be successful in helping others think about their careers. Becoming familiar with this next tool will also increase its usefulness when you use it to help others start to think about what is important to them in a career.

Integral to the process of career planning is having a real understanding of yourself; what motivates and what inspires you and what does not. Your life experiences, your principles and values, your relationships with family, friends and colleagues and professional identity influence your career choices. Therefore, the greater your self-awareness the more satisfying your career choices could be.

Your ethics set the boundaries as to how far you are prepared to go to get what you want. Work values are personal to you too. You will be happiest and most fulfilled in a job that incorporates your main work values.

Eight career anchor categories have been identified by Schein to increase people's insights into their strengths and motivation as part of career development: these are technical or functional competence, general managerial competence, autonomy or independence, security or stability, entrepreneurial creativity, service or dedication to a cause, pure challenge and lifestyle.[11] People define their self-image in terms of these traits, and come to understand more about their talents, motives and values – and which of these they would not give up if forced to make a choice.

Nature of career anchors

Career anchors help you to understand the meaning and implications of past career decisions and inform future ones, whether or not you work in the health service. They give a clearer understanding of:

- your orientations towards work
- your motives
- your values
- your talents.

Career anchors will help you to:

- define the themes and patterns that are dominant in your life
- understand your own approach to work and career
- identify and clarify your talents
- provide reasons for career choices
- take action to secure a fulfilling career.

The questions listed in Table 6.1 will help you to identify your career anchors and prompt you to consider your areas of competence, values and motivation. Read through the detailed descriptions that follow and then come back to complete the box. Fill in the middle column rating how important you perceive each career anchor to be for you. Then complete the right-hand column gauging how you rate each career anchor in respect of the main job you currently hold. Add another column or two if you have a portfolio of other jobs and you want to think about each individually with a separate column for each.

Table 6.1: Identify your career anchors and how well you perceive these to match your current job

Schein career anchor[11]	How important is this aspect of your career to you (score out of 5 where 0 is nil and 5 is a great deal)?	How does this match with your current situation (score out of 5 where 0 is nil and 5 is a great deal)?
Technical or functional competence		
Managerial competence		
Autonomy or independence		
Security or stability		
Entrepreneurial or creative		
Service or dedication to a cause		
Pure challenge		
Lifestyle		

Is there a mismatch between what career anchors you rate as being most important for you and those that relate to your current situation?

Career anchor descriptions

Technical and functional competence

A high score in this area suggests that you value being able to apply your skills and to develop those skills to an ever higher level.

General managerial competence

A high score in this area suggests that you value the opportunity to climb to a high enough level to enable you to integrate the efforts of others across functions and to be responsible for the output of a particular unit in your trust or practice, or other organisation. You want to be responsible and accountable for total results, and you identify your own work with the success of the organisation for which you work.

Autonomy and independence

A high score in this area suggests that you value being able to define your own work in your own way. You want to remain in jobs that allow you flexibility regarding how and when you work.

Security and stability

A high score in this area suggests that you value employment security or tenure in a job or organisation or financial security. People anchored in this way are *always* concerned with these issues and build their entire self-image around security and stability.

Entrepreneurial creativity

A high score in this area suggests that you value the opportunity to create an organisation or enterprise of your own, built on your own abilities and your willing-ness to take risks and to overcome obstacles.

Service and dedication to a cause

A high score in this area suggests that you appreciate being able to pursue work that achieves something in keeping with your values and beliefs.

Pure challenge

A high score in this area suggests that you value the opportunity to work on solutions to challenging or seemingly unsolvable problems, or to overcome difficult obstacles.

Lifestyle

A high score in this area suggests that you value being able to balance and integrate your personal needs, family needs and the requirements of your career.

Discover your hidden talents

Make time for career planning. Take stock and review your career to date. Evaluate your strengths and skills and decide what you want to do, to continue in your current path or diversify to parallel or alternative fields. Then, taking account of the oppor-tunities on offer and any circumstances limiting your choice of actions, push on with your career development and achieve your career goals.[12,13] And take the final challenge, *see* Box 6.7.

Box 6.7:   The challenge is to create your vision for your beautiful career[14]

So where are you now?
What are you proud of in your personal life and job?
What can you celebrate?
What would you like to be different?

References

1   Chambers R (ed) (2005) *Career Planning for Everyone in the NHS: your toolkit*. Radcliffe Publishing, Oxford.

2   Chambers R, Cobb S, Mohanna K, Roberts M and Thornett A (2003) *Improving the Quality of Careers Information and Guidance in Primary Care*. Staffordshire University, Stafford.

3   Chambers R, Mohanna K and Field S (2000) *Opportunities and Options in Medical Careers*. Radcliffe Medical Press, Oxford.

4   Houghton A (2004) Leaving your job: part 1. *BMJ Careers*. **6 March:** 93–4.

5   Chambers R, Mohanna K and Chambers S (2003) *Survival Skills for Doctors and their Families*. Radcliffe Medical Press, Oxford.

6   Chambers R (1999) *Survival Skills for GPs*. Radcliffe Medical Press, Oxford.

7   British Medical Association (2004) *BMA Cohort Study of 1995 Medical Graduates*. Ninth report. Health Policy and Economic Research Unit, BMA, London.

8   Mohanna K and Chambers R (2003) Career crises. *BMJ Career Focus*. **326:** s35–6.

9   The National Institute for Careers Education and Counselling (NICEC) (2003) *Informing Choices*. NICEC, Careers Research and Advisory Centre (CRAC), London.

10   Maslow AH (1970) *Motivation and Personality*. Harper and Row, New York.

11   Schein E (1996) *Career Anchors, Discovering your Real Values*. Pfeiffer, Oxford.

12   Learndirect (2003) *Discover your Hidden Talents*. The Open University, Milton Keynes. www.learndirect-advice.co.uk (accessed 9 August 2005).

13   Langdon K (2004) *Cultivate a Cool Career*. Infinite Ideas, Oxford.

14   MacDonald R (2003) *My Beautiful Career. BMJ Careers Workbook*. BMJcareers, London. bmjcareers.com (accessed 9 August 2005).

7

Talking about careers as an appraiser

Kay Mohanna

This chapter is about the specific knowledge, skills and beliefs you require to talk about career planning as an appraiser. You will inevitably find that many of these attributes are the same ones you need to be an effective appraiser, whatever the subject under discussion. For that matter they may well be the same interpersonal skills that you use in other aspects of your professional roles, either working with colleagues or with patients.

Appraisal has been in place in industry, commerce and the public sectors for decades. In the NHS, health professionals, managers and administrative staff are now all expected to undergo annual appraisals. In England, appraisal became a contractual requirement for all hospital consultants from April 2001, and for GPs of all types of contractual status by April 2004.

A definition of appraisal that encapsulates the developmental purpose of appraisal is:

> A professional process of constructive dialogue in which the (person) being appraised has a formal structured opportunity to reflect on his or her work and to consider how his or her effectiveness might be improved.[1]

This definition reflects the widely accepted view that appraisal should be a formative process that is concerned with the professional development and personal fulfilment of the doctor being appraised, leading to an improvement in their performance at work. It is very likely then, that in your role as an appraiser you will be involved in conversations with doctors being appraised, who are considering their career options and development. They may be asking themselves if they are happy at work, whether their circumstances dictate a change, or whether the time has come to seek a new challenge.

In any organisation the aims of an effective appraisal scheme are:

- to give individuals feedback on their performance
- to explore the limits of existing knowledge and skills – of individuals or teams
- to offer a systematic development needs analysis process for all members of staff
- to produce PDPs that establish how training and development needs will be met.

For the appraiser, there will always be a balance between helping the individual make the most of him/herself and helping the organisation (practice, department or trust) to make the most effective use of its employees.

In North Stoke teaching primary care trust the definition of appraisal explicitly includes the opportunity to include talking about future career planning (*see* Box 7.1).

Box 7.1:   Career planning is part of appraisal[2]

Employee appraisal is:

- an opportunity to stimulate you through praise and encouragement
- a chance to reflect
- a chance to discuss any problem areas
- a brainstorming session on your working relationships
- a chance to consider your future career plans
- the opportunity to identify and plan training and development needs and opportunities.

Employee appraisal is *not*:

- a substitute for the disciplinary procedure
- an opportunity to list all your gripes from the previous year
- an opportunity to belittle a member of staff or put them in their place
- a chance for a manager/appraiser to tell a member of staff what they need to do for the next 12 months.

The format of appraisals for doctors follows the sequence of headings in *Good Medical Practice*.[3] Considering these headings can show you how you may find yourself in a discussion about career choices at any stage of the appraisal.

Good clinical care and maintaining good medical practice

Here the appraisee is encouraged to reflect on the type of clinical care they are engaged in. Questions to encourage that reflection include:

- what do you think are the main strengths and weaknesses of your clinical practice?
- what do you think are your clinical care development needs for the future?
- what factors in your workplace, or more widely, constrain you significantly in achieving what you aim for in your clinical work?
- what professional or personal factors significantly constrain you in maintaining and developing your skills and knowledge?
- (and more explicitly) how do you see your job and career developing over the next few years?

Any one of these questions could prompt a discussion around whether the doctor being appraised feels constrained by their current situation from practising as they had aspired to do when they started out in medicine. As they think about the audits they have done and the work involved in developing protocols, they may realise that they are not spending time on the kinds of cases that interest them. They may start to feel that their current job gets in the way of them being the kind of professional that they set out to be. The final two questions might enable them to see that there are specific, remediable factors that are getting in the way of this, and they might choose to address them.

Relationships with patients

For this category appraisers often ask the question:

- what do you think are the strengths and weaknesses of your relationships with patients?

An answer that suggests serious interpersonal difficulties raises issues around developing a career away from a focus on clinical practice to laboratory-based or research jobs, for instance. Likewise a colleague with good interpersonal skills may feel that a move to a job or role with more patient contact might be more rewarding. For doctors in training who are being appraised, these questions, accompanied by suitable, robust exercises to help determine the real nature of their relationships with patients, can have a serious impact on career choices that they make.

Working with colleagues

Questioning in this area can precipitate some self disclosures that would never have been discussed before the advent of appraisal. Appraisees should be asked to consider:

- what do you think are the main strengths and weaknesses of your relationships with colleagues?

Some appraisees might be unhappy at work because of the people that they work with. Others rely on their colleagues to get them through the working day. Questions in this category can help appraisees contemplating a career change realise that it is more likely a clash of personalities within their current workplace that is at the bottom of their difficulties rather than the nature of the job itself.

An appraisal discussion might address the appraisee's preferred role in a team and their strengths as a leader. These insights might uncover the reasons for dysfunctional working relationships and might suggest how they could be deployed more fruitfully at work.

Teaching and training, and research

Not everyone being appraised will document activity in these areas. For those that do, ask them to consider these questions:

- what factors constrain you in developing as a teacher?
- would you like to do more teaching or training?
- how would you appraise the quality or purpose of any research work that you do?
- what are the constraints to you undertaking teaching or training or research?

A doctor in general practice might aspire to training practice status but work with others who see training as a chore that limits his or her ambition to be a trainer. With the growth in opportunities for established doctors to develop portfolio careers, it might be possible to address a desire to teach by negotiating a change in hours and searching for a parallel teaching position, perhaps in a local university or for the trust training and education department. It might be possible to change the minds of others in the team or department, if time could be spent on investigating the implications and advantages of gaining training status or experience.

Undertaking research is less common in the community than the secondary care sector, but opportunities and funding for being involved in research do exist. Appraisees may need careers guidance and information to see that they can become involved in research on a part-time basis, without it necessitating a major change in their career.

Management activity

Many doctors did not anticipate the level of management activity they would be engaged with when they started their training. For others, the chance to be involved in decision making and policy and strategy development is a welcome opportunity.

All doctors should be asked:

- describe any management activities you undertake that are not related to your clinical practice or department in which you work
- how would you describe your success in these areas?
- what are the constraints?

Their responses might give you the opportunity as an appraiser to help them to think about the balance in their week between management and other activities, and whether they want to address and renegotiate this balance.

Health

This is a very important category for any doctor to address, but especially for those who may be undergoing some form of career crisis. Appraisees should be asked:

- do you feel there are any health-related issues for you that may put patients at risk? Please mention any problems or concerns raised during the year and any steps you feel should be taken to safeguard the position.

Appraisees may be reluctant to address aspects of this category. You may need all your skills of empathy and tact to tease out any problems. Its presence as an appraisal-form category does give a starting point for discussion. Ill-health can both result from and cause problems in a person's work and career. Alcoholism, stress, mental illness and physical disability are all issues that might bring about a career crisis, while at the same time removing some of the coping mechanisms through which good career choices are usually made. You will need all your diplomacy as an appraiser in order to make the most of the opportunity to move beyond a standard 'everything is fine' answer.

Appraisers as givers of careers information, advice or guidance

You may feel that you are not well equipped to be giving careers information, advice or guidance. You may even feel that it is not your place. However as an appraiser you will be able to bring to the conversation many factors that can help a colleague who may be struggling with issues about a possible change in career.

As an appraiser you know that your role is to help facilitate the thinking of a colleague so that they can reflect on where they are and where they want to be. In terms of *careers information giving*, you may feel that your role is to be no more than a signpost to other sources of information that can help them to consider their options. So to be an effective appraiser in this aspect requires a basic level of knowledge about sources of help, should they be required. It is possible that your role in this aspect of careers planning is just to say, 'have you thought about asking ... about this?'

The domain of *careers advice or guidance* is the one in which many appraisers will find themselves, and feel comfortable taking up the challenge. This role sits well within the definition of appraisal as being a process of facilitated self-reflection.

Colleagues who require the level of support of *career counselling* may be really struggling and have got to the position where they can no longer see the wood for the trees. You may be able to clarify issues for them or help them to define the problem explicitly. It is unlikely that you will have the time or expertise they need to give them in-depth support, and you will need to signpost them to an expert careers counsellor. They may have become depressed or have distorted perceptions that get in the way of them thinking clearly and making rational decisions. Your main role again here might be to advise them to access sources of further help, such as their own GP or an occupational health service.

Many appraisers have come to the job by virtue of being a line manager or lead for a doctor in their organisation, such as medical or unit directors. Others, such as in GP appraisal, have applied for the job through a desire to help colleagues, and will have been selected for the post because of their good interpersonal skills amongst other aspects. One thing both of these routes is likely to lack is any specific training in providing careers advice or guidance. How prepared do you currently feel to take on that role? Consider the following list of activities in Table 7.1 that can be required when talking to others about their careers.[4] From the list identify two categories in which you feel least skilled. Then consider the two in which you feel most skilled. Consider the implications of this and how you might apply that knowledge.

Table 7.1: Range of approaches when talking to others about their careers

	Implication	*Application*
Giving advice – offering suggestions		
Offering information		
Challenging what is said to you		
Helping another person to express emotion		
Drawing another person out		
Encouraging and supporting another person		

Careers advice or guidance in the appraisal conversation

So, imagine that you are in the middle of an appraisal when it becomes apparent that careers guidance is called for. Your appraisee admits to being unhappy with their job and thinks it might be the direction of their career that is the problem. Maybe, they suggest, it's time for a change. You will want to help them to identify the actual focus for their dissatisfaction. Otherwise, they may try to change the parts of their life they feel they have the power to change – which may not address the real problem, and have triggered unnecessary change. They may switch career only to find that the problem 'follows them'.

Typical mid-career reflections can be brought into the open by asking:

• are you unsure about your future career direction?
• do you believe you could achieve more?
• do you want to take control of your career?
• are you facing change – in your personal circumstances, in the NHS?
• which aspects do you want to change?
• what kind of work do you enjoy?
• what transferable skills do you have?
• how does your current work measure up to your inner values?

Then ask about the work itself:

• what sort of people do you want to care for – the ages and kinds of patients?
• what sort of people do you want to work with – small team or big organisation?
• where do you want to work – in the community or hospital, rural or urban?

Appraisees will need to ask themselves:

• what will happen to my income?
• how will I cope with the further training – hours, practical difficulties, examinations?
• what opportunities are there for me to progress?

And you will want to guide them to consider:

• will I be out of the frying pan into the fire?
• can I balance this job with my commitments outside medicine?
• will there be opportunities for parallel career interests – research, writing, education, consultancy, private work or work-related hobbies?

You will need to make a decision. Are you and the appraisee able to rationally discuss the pros and cons of their situation, or is it possible that they are depressed or otherwise ill? If these or other barriers to reflection are present it may be that they need referral elsewhere for help, such as to their GP, occupational health services or for career counselling. However you and your appraisee may agree to spend some time looking at the issues involved.

Summary

You can facilitate another person's smooth journey towards a change in their career by ensuring that they identify specific causes for their dissatisfaction with their present situation, so they have a clear idea of what a good change would look like. Any plan to swap career tracks should only be made after an analysis of personal attributes and aspirations, to try to predict what changes need to be made. It may be that the causes of the unhappiness are not issues that are directly related to the career at all. Having decided to make changes, it is important that they be mapped out with an action plan that has clear objectives and staged steps to measure the progress towards the target. Potential pitfalls or barriers should also be identified in advance, and contingency plans be built in. The skills needed to facilitate this as an appraiser are the same ones as those you use in activities such as planning and developing a PDP with an appraisee. Since these are core skills of appraising, providing careers advice and guidance fits well with the role of an appraiser.

References

1 Kendall L and Lissauer R (2003) *The Future Health Worker.* Institute for Public Policy Research, London.

2 North Stoke Primary Care Trust (2003) *Definition of Appraisal.* North Stoke Primary Care Trust, Staffordshire.

3 General Medical Council (2003) *Good Medical Practice.* General Medical Council, London.

4 Chambers R, Mohanna K and Field S (2000). *Opportunities and Options in Medical Careers.* Radcliffe Medical Press, Oxford.

8

Techniques and tools for being an effective provider of careers information, advice and guidance

Ruth Chambers and Kay Mohanna

One way to describe the knowledge and skills you will need for your role and responsibilities as providing careers information, advice or guidance to medical students or doctors is the *NHS Knowledge and Skills Framework* (KSF).[1] This framework seems to be an appropriate tool for describing the characteristics of any employed post in the NHS, and is part of the NHS *Agenda for Change* initiative.[2] Under *Agenda for Change*, the majority of staff employed by the NHS will be placed in one of eight pay bands depending on the knowledge, responsibility, skills and effort needed for their job.[2] The NHS KSF is intended to be used as part of a structured approach to training, development and review, with the overall aim of improving consistency and quality of services to patients. The six core dimensions and 22 specific dimensions of the KSF are based on what knowledge and skills staff are currently expected to possess. Adopting the KSF will have significant implications for revealing previously unfilled and/or unrecognised training needs for all those using the framework.

Each dimension of the NHS KSF is further described in levels, climbing from Level 1 to Level 4. Each level describes successively more advanced knowledge and skills and/ or increasing complexity of application of knowledge and skills to the demands of work. The content of each level builds on that of the preceding one.[1]

Turn back to Box 5.2 (page 47) to review a brief description of the six core dimensions of the knowledge and skills as relevant to someone providing careers information, advice or guidance to medical students or doctors.[1]

You might be able to demonstrate that you are competent in providing careers information, advice or guidance by referring to evidence of your knowledge and skills matched against the list of competencies in Tables 8.1 to 8.5, but that does not ensure that you perform consistently well. One of the downsides of tools and frameworks such as the NHS KSF is that they imply that performance can be anticipated and measured, whereas in reality in healthcare it is difficult to do so in a complex and changing health setting.

Performing consistently well will depend on your personal application and morale as someone providing careers information, advice or guidance, the availability of resources and support such as training and protected time, and the expectations and preparedness of those being advised. It is not sufficient to have knowledge and know how (competence) but you also need to apply those knowledge and skills in practice as consistently good performance in action.[3] As a careers adviser you need to possess high order professional judgement as well as the core competencies to be *able to apply* your knowledge and skills consistently in appropriate ways, with the range of people with whom you are working. You will have many attributes relating to the KSF over and above those described by Tables 8.1 to 8.5, to be competent to deal with complex situations that may crop up between you and those you advise in considering their professional or personal experiences.

We have set out the tools and techniques that will be useful to you for developing your knowledge and skills, under the six headings of the relevant dimensions of the NHS KSF (*see* Box 5.2). You should read through our descriptions of what each dimension of knowledge and skills might entail. Then consider how your own knowledge and skills match up. If you have a learning need, we offer several alternative ways by which you might build your knowledge and skills or positive attitude for that specific dimension.

This should be useful for your own personal development and careers advice portfolio(s). Various types of audit, feedback from colleagues, peers and those you are advising, comparison with best practice, critical incident analysis (e.g. a complaint from someone you have advised) are all good methods of gathering objective evidence.

Consistently practise good communication skills[4,5]

Effective communication skills in providing careers information, advice or guidance might entail:

- understanding and applying good interpersonal communication: recognising and taking account of the other person's favoured interpersonal style in order to optimise communication between you both; summarising what the other person says, to check that you are both on the same wavelength
- using active listening
- using supportive non-verbal body language, reading verbal and non-verbal signals of those you are advising
- establishing rapport, being able to create a suitable atmosphere, putting others at ease
- giving constructive feedback
- recognising and sensitively managing areas of resistance and conflict within the career discussion process, managing any anger or aggression
- skills: influencing, assertiveness, facilitation
- challenging assumptions and statements of those you are advising, as appropriate
- enabling a constructive outcome to the career discussion: judging when further detail is needed, effective summarisation and clarification
- having an enthusiastic and positive attitude to careers information, advice or guidance
- maintaining confidentiality consistent with legislation and NHS policies
- establishing the help that others require, and acting on this appropriately: knowing about career pathways and systems, knowing what trusts or other primary care organisations can do to help, identifying resource needs.

Consider the extent to which you (i) have the knowledge and skills, and (ii) practise them – during careers information or advice sessions and in your everyday working life in other aspects of your job (you might generalise the items in the list above to 'colleague or member of staff'). Complete your audit checklist in Table 8.1.

How expert are you?

Think how expert you are for each aspect of effective communication that we have listed in the left hand column of Table 8.1 (look back to Chapter 5 to review the approach from the novice to expert spectrum of competency).

- *Aware?* If you are merely 'aware', you might be aware that the particular knowledge and/or skill is important and have undertaken some preliminary reading and learning, but are not yet confident, practised or skilled in employing that feature of effective communication.
- *Competent?* If you are 'competent' you will have a good basic knowledge and be skilled in communicating with a typical person whom you advise about their career.
- *Expert?* If you are an 'expert' you will have an enormous range of experience and intuitive grasp of situations. You will be able to interpret and synthesise information and handle a wide range of communication problems in different contexts.[6]

How frequently do you use that aspect of effective communication?

Think how often you employ that feature of effective communication with others at work. Think more widely than the giving of careers information or advice, and of your interactions with colleagues of all levels of seniority and patients. Is it at least daily or at least weekly or at least monthly with your colleagues or others at work? The more such knowledge and skills are part of your normal behaviour, the more likely they will feature naturally and consistently in the way you discuss others' careers.

Make your assessment more objective

Seek others' views of your competence or performance in relation to effective communication. You might simply ask someone else who knows you well to complete a second copy of the audit in Table 8.1 and compare your pre-completed table with their perspective of you – and of course discuss any differences with them so that you can learn from their input. You might seek feedback from the person you advise about their career, or others for whom you have a role or responsibility such as in line management, educational supervision, mentoring or coaching.

Table 8.1: Self-check of own knowledge and skills in respect of communication between you and students or doctors whom you inform or advise about their careers

Aspect of communication	How expert are you? Aware? Competent? Expert?	How frequently do you use these? At least: every day? weekly? monthly?
Understanding and applying good interpersonal communication, active listening		
Establishing rapport with those you advise about their career		
Using non-verbal body language		
Giving constructive feedback		
Recognising and managing conflict		
Challenge others' beliefs constructively		
Skills: influencing, assertiveness, facilitation		
Enabling a constructive outcome to a career discussion		
Having an enthusiastic attitude to career development		
Maintaining confidentiality		
Establishing help the other person requires		

General tips for improving your communication skills

We all think that we know about communication skills – and are often baffled when someone misinterprets something that we have said or done. No-one should be complacent that they cannot improve their communication skills.

You can learn how to observe, evaluate and change how you communicate with other people. Receiving feedback from others helps to make the necessary changes. Understand not just what is said but the feelings behind the words. Consider the verbal and non-verbal aspects of communication, as described in Figure 8.1.

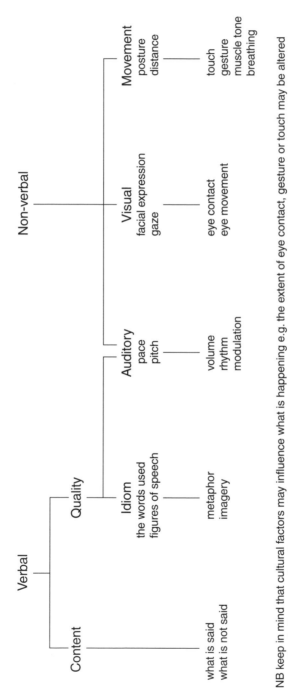

Figure 8.1: Signs of the mental state in communication.

The meaning of language[4,5]

Most of the time you understand what people say, but sometimes your 'wires get crossed'. Some examples of poor language skills are:

- *taking things literally*: the answer to 'Have you seen that file I put down?' is not 'Yes', but 'It's over there on the table'
- *action meanings*: people often use action statements when they do not like to ask directly for things. Saying 'It's very fresh in here with the window open' can be a request for the window to be shut, and the speaker will be quite offended if you reply 'Yes, it's nice to have fresh air coming in'
- *connotative meanings*: these can suggest emotions but express what is said and what is meant differently. Many people remember their full name being used when someone was telling them off. People who use metaphors implying that the workplace is a war zone (e.g. we will attack this problem on several fronts and defend our position on this matter) may be expressing their inner feelings about it being a battlefield
- *Using jargon*: the use of jargon can sometimes be an unconscious attempt to prevent communication and understanding – after all if you do not understand what I am talking about you cannot possibly do my job! More often it is failure to use feedback (or lack of it) to modify what is being said to the level of understanding of the listener
- *Using formal or informal styles in the wrong settings*: people speak differently to their friends than to colleagues, or to people at work with whom they have an unequal power relationship. Generally, the more formal the event, the more formal the language, and some people find it difficult to gauge the right level. Cultural factors affect the situation – what might seem excessively formal to an American, may seem over casual to someone from Japan.

More general tips for improving your skills for good interpersonal communication are given in Box 8.1.

Box 8.1:   Skills for good interpersonal communication[5]

1 Listen with genuine interest
2 Create a conducive environment
3 Be encouraging
4 Show understanding and empathy
5 Check current understanding
6 Reflect/summarise and paraphrase answers
7 Use closed questions for exploration
8 Use open questions for clarification
9 Adopt a similar language and avoid jargon
10 Use plural pronouns to indicate partnership
11 Be provisional rather than dogmatic
12 Be descriptive not judgemental
13 Comment on the issues rather then personalities
14 Encourage eye contact
15 Give information in clear simple terms and use repetition
16 Check understanding
17 Use silence

The difference between hearing and listening: use active listening

The quality of your attention when discussing careers with a medical student or doctor is achieved by a concentrated form of listening. There is a great deal of difference between *hearing* and *listening*. Hearing is a passive activity, while listening is active and requires you to *show* that you have been listening. There is a real difference between the listening which takes place with a patient, when taking a case history, and the kind of listening you will need when helping a colleague to reflect on their career or personal situation. When taking a case history you are assessing what they say with a view to making a diagnosis. The first step with those you advise is to enable them to express themselves fully and feel understood. This process consists of reflecting back what has been said, paraphrasing and summarising at frequent intervals.

Only when someone feels certain that they are understood will they proceed to share their thoughts and feelings. That should help the individuals you are advising about their careers to move forward to thinking about the future and drawing up plans for action.

Exploring

Try to use open questions to expand the conversation that encourage the other person to describe information and explore or reflect upon their feelings. Avoid using 'Why?' questions as they tend to trigger defensive responses. Instead, ask 'What?', 'How?' and 'When?' to draw out the person you advising.

Creating rapport

Rapport is the process of building and sustaining a relationship of mutual trust and understanding. It is the ability to relate to others, in a way that makes people feel at their ease. When you have rapport with someone, you feel at ease, conversation flows and silences are easy. It is the basis of good communication and is a form of influence. It is a major component of listening, when the whole body indicates interest in what the other person is saying.

Building rapport is a technique described and practised in neurolinguistic programming (NLP), which is the study of what works in thinking, language and behaviour.[7] You might use NLP to enable those you appraise to plan ahead after identifying their learning and service development needs. NLP is based on a simple model of goal achievement set out as four stages:

- decide what you want
- do something
- notice what happens
- be flexible – be prepared to change.

Steps in creating rapport and relationship building[4,5]

- You should be aware of yourself and your 'body language'. Make a conscious effort to match or mirror as many of the other person's characteristics as possible: posture and the position of your body, legs, arms, hands and fingers, and how your head and shoulders are held, your expression.
- Ensure that you make and keep sufficient eye contact (too much is intimidating).
- Voice: think about the pace, volume, and intonation of your voice. Listen to the type of words being used by those you advise. Try to use a similar voice and words.
- Create an environment that facilitates rapport and easy conversation: for example, seating position, dress, décor of room etc.
- Be friendly and attentive, and adopt an informal style.
- Use plural pronouns to indicate partnership as appropriate, though not to imply that you as the careers adviser are taking responsibility for the actions of those you advise.
- Use self-disclosure about your own fears or experiences to establish trust and common ground (but not too often as the session is focused on the other person's agenda, not yours).
- Make comments that are provisional rather than dogmatic, inviting discussion. Comment on the problem rather than making judgements.
- Ask open rather than closed questions.
- Listen actively and reflectively.
- Pick up and follow themes that those you are advising about their careers introduce.
- Use clear, relevant and brief communication, rather than rambling anecdotes. It is the other person's agenda that is important in the careers discussion. You should resist any temptation to indulge yourself by enjoying reciting your own career experiences for your own benefit, unless you are describing a relevant model of career progression.
- Learn to recognise and interpret and use your own feelings, so that you do not relay these inappropriately to those whom you are advising.

Remembering the JoHari window model

The JoHari window is a useful model for thinking about communication.[8] It will help you to understand the function of feedback and the way you and others relate to each other by interpersonal activity, identifying strengths and learning needs. Box 8.2 illustrates the concept. The four panes of the 'window', or four quadrants, represent how relationships are built up by an accumulation of information from 'self' and 'others' – in this case you and the student or doctor with whom you are discussing their career development.

Consider the crossed lines that separate the four quadrants as if they can be moved to vary the size of the four quadrants in Box 8.2 to those of Box 8.3. The horizontal line represents 'exposure' (that is, extent of self-disclosure) and the vertical line represents feedback. By such exposure, those being advised open up, share ideas and information, and talk about their feelings and opinions. As they increase exposure, their 'façade' decreases, but the 'blind-spot' may increase through less time being given to feedback.

Focusing on giving constructive feedback may increase the façade as it allows less time for 'exposure' for people you appraise to disclose their feelings and fears.

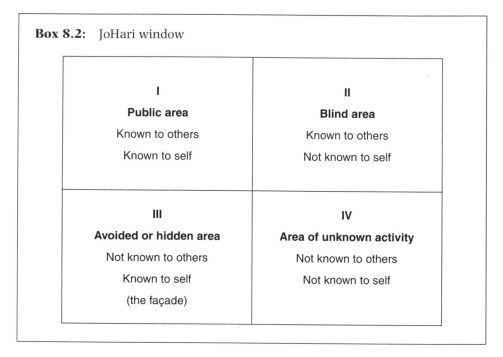

Box 8.2: JoHari window

I **Public area** Known to others Known to self	**II** **Blind area** Known to others Not known to self
III **Avoided or hidden area** Not known to others Known to self (the façade)	**IV** **Area of unknown activity** Not known to others Not known to self

When you and the person you are advising do not know each other very well, the area in quadrant I is small and quadrant III is large, as in Box 8.3.

Box 8.3: JoHari window for new relationships

I **Public area** Known to others Known to self	**II** **Blind area** Known to others Not known to self
III **Avoided or hidden area** Not known to others Known to self (the façade)	**IV** **Area of unknown activity** Not known to others Not known to self

As you get to know the person you are advising better, quadrant III shrinks in size and quadrant I enlarges. Poor communication between you and the other person inhibits the enlargement of quadrant I. The quadrants on the right, especially quadrant II, are susceptible to feedback from you and others, and reducing this area increases the other person's awareness of his or her strengths and careers needs.

Challenge from you or from the colleagues of individuals being advised, or other external factors reduces the size of quadrant IV and increases the sizes of quadrants I and II. A person's internal monitoring also helps to reduce the size of quadrant IV, so that their qualities, skills, or abilities in this area can become uncovered and recognised, then moved to quadrants I or III.

There is universal curiosity about quadrants III and IV, but this is held in check by custom, social training and fear of what might be revealed. You need to be sensitive about the covert content of the blind-spot, the façade and the hidden area in quadrants II, III and IV, and respect others' privacy about information kept hidden for reasons of social training or custom. Up to a point, the larger the area called the arena in the top left quadrant in Box 8.3, the more productive the relationship is likely to be.

You might categorise individuals you advise about their careers into one of four types of people using this JoHari window model:

- *Type A*: little exposure, little feedback seeking. This type of person is often perceived as withdrawn, aloof or impersonal, where the unknown square (in Boxes 8.2 or 8.3) is the largest. This may induce resentment in others who may take the behaviour personally. It is common in large bureaucratic organisations.
- *Type B*: increased feedback seeking, little exposure. These people decrease the information about themselves available to others, whilst requiring more from others, either through fear or a wish for power or control. Others may react by withdrawing trust or becoming hostile.
- *Type C*: increased exposure, neglect of feedback. These people are oblivious to the impact they have on others. They have a large blind-spot as the opportunity for feedback is rare. They may be confident of their own opinions and insensitive, with little concern for the feelings of others. Listeners may become angry and reluctant to tell them anything.
- *Type D*: balanced. These people have a large arena as feedback-seeking and exposure behaviours are well used. They are open and candid. Initially others may be put on the defensive, but once these people are seen as genuine, then productive relationships can follow. They induce an open balanced response in others.

Building trust and relationships

Trust requires two things: competency and caring. Competency alone or caring by itself will not create trust. Scholtes[9] believes that if you think someone is competent, but you do not think that they care about you or the things that are important to you, you will respect them but not necessarily trust them – *see* Figure 8.2. On the other hand, if you think someone cares about you but you do not feel they are competent or capable, you will have affection for that person but not necessarily trust them to do the job in hand.

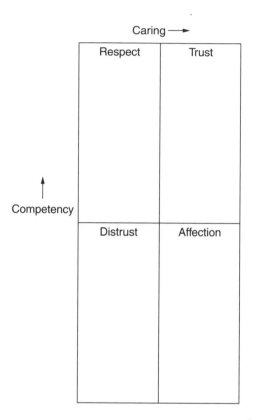

Figure 8.2:   Scholtes' relationship of competency and caring to trust.[9]

You can encourage people to trust you if you:

- do what you say you will do and do not make promises you cannot or will not keep
- listen to people carefully and tell them what you think they are saying. People trust others when they believe that they understand them
- understand what matters to people. People trust those who they believe are looking out for their best interests.

You can encourage good relationships with people if you:

- are able to talk to each other and are willing to listen to each other
- respect each other and show this in ways that the other person wants
- know each other well enough to understand and respect the other person's values and beliefs
- do not hide your shortcomings. This may improve your image but does not build trust
- do not confuse trustworthiness with friendship. Trust does not automatically come with friendship
- tell the truth! Be honest.

Giving constructive feedback[10,11]

Constructive feedback is the art of holding conversations with others about their performance, and it has two elements: it should contain enough specific detail and advice to enable the recipient to reflect and enhance their practice, and it should be positive and supportive in tone. Effective feedback has an impact not only on the learning process but also gives messages to others about their effectiveness and worth, and contributes to building their self-esteem.

It is important that as well as being positive in tone, you should balance your commentary between areas to improve and feedback that is positive in content. You should aim to give feedback about their apparent deficiencies *and* strengths. To see why this is so, consider the model of the development of expertise in Figure 8.3.

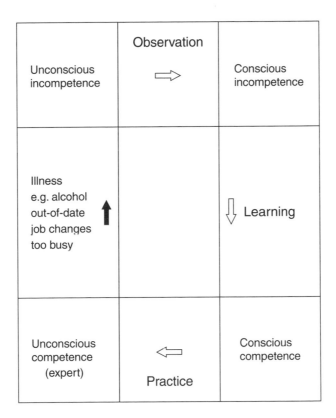

Figure 8.3:   The importance of feedback in the development of expertise (competency cycle).

Starting in the top left-hand quadrant in Figure 8.3, you are blissfully unaware of your shortcomings until something happens to make you aware of them. That might be the realisation, when you start working with patients, that the education you had at university was not appropriate, and that you are out of your depth. It could be a patient complaint or adverse incident or it could be feedback from a line manager, tutor or colleague.

This realisation is a painful process, often referred to as cognitive dissonance, but until you become aware you cannot start the process of learning. Remember it's when you feel uncomfortable that you are just about to learn something. Too much discomfort however can be demotivating, and some people might give up at this stage if they feel there is too much to learn or they will never be good enough. Some feedback about their other strengths would thus be supportive at this stage.

The process of learning, with all that that entails, can then proceed and you will master the new understanding, knowledge or task. You reach a stage where you know something new or know how to do something and can perform competently, so long as circumstances remain constant – as represented by the bottom right quadrant of Figure 8.3. With practice and experience you then become expert. You can apply and modify your knowledge and skills in new situations that you may never have met before. At this stage, the bottom left quadrant, you could teach others. It is also the stage when, through familiarity, you can lose sight of your strengths, as your skills become automatic. Feedback on performance at this stage needs to include things you are good at so that you do not accept them as commonplace, you can reflect on them, keep them up to date and highlight them. In some ways, feedback needs to take you from left to right across the bottom of the competency cycle to make you aware of your expertise again so that you can effectively teach others.

It is possible to move back to unconscious incompetence from the position of expertise, in the direction of the bold arrow, through severe mental illness for example, or degenerative disease without insight, or even failure to keep up to date. Feedback in this position is very likely to be difficult, another good reason to include a reminder of remaining skills and positive attributes. (This model has some similarities with the JoHari window – *see* Boxes 8.2 and 8.3, which describes balanced communication between feedback seeking and self-disclosure to minimise either the areas of hidden information in a relationship or lack of insight.)

The skill of the effective careers adviser is to find the balance between support and challenge, and the best feedback is high on both support and challenge. Figure 8.4 describes the qualities of feedback of different dimensions.

There is one golden rule for giving constructive feedback: give positive praise of things that have been well done first. Some general rules are:

1 focus on behaviour rather than interpretation
2 give specific examples
3 aim to be descriptive or sensory based rather than interpretive, non-sensory based
4 aim to be non-judgemental rather than evaluative.

Read up elsewhere on different models of giving feedback.[11]

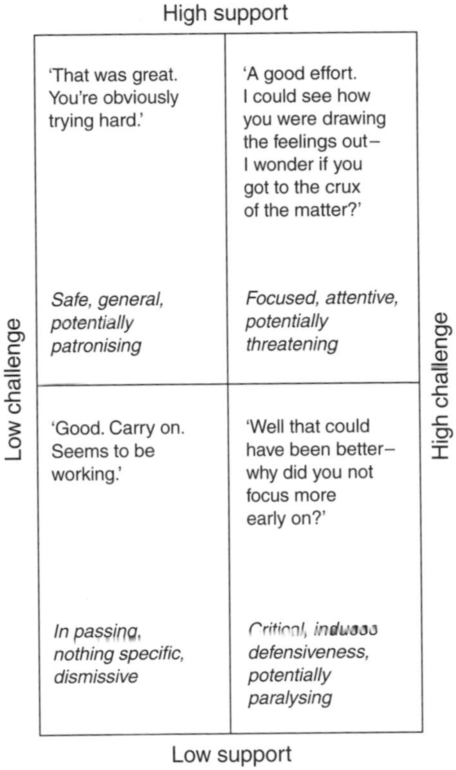

High support

'That was great. You're obviously trying hard.'	'A good effort. I could see how you were drawing the feelings out— I wonder if you got to the crux of the matter?'
Safe, general, potentially patronising	*Focused, attentive, potentially threatening*
'Good. Carry on. Seems to be working.'	'Well that could have been better— why did you not focus more early on?'
In passing, nothing specific, dismissive	*Critical, induces defensiveness, potentially paralysing*

Low challenge ← → High challenge

Low support

Figure 8.4: Qualities of feedback in relation to extent of support and challenge.

Develop your own skills and knowledge and provide information and advice to others to help their development

This means developing your own and others' knowledge, skills and practice by:

- understanding the healthcare context relevant to those you are advising about their careers, and making realistic allowances for problems and issues (including your and their attitudes, beliefs, learning styles, motivation etc)
- understanding national and local healthcare priorities and how these are relevant to your and the circumstances of those you advise
- evaluating the currency and sufficiency of your own knowledge and practice in providing careers information, advice or guidance
- developing more in-depth knowledge and skills in careers information, advice or guidance as an integral part of a PDP
- being able to recognise and acknowledge whether discussion and learning has addressed the career development needs of the person concerned

- working with others (including those you are advising about their careers) to develop, identify and implement appropriate learning opportunities within and outside work
- negotiating and encouraging goal setting and action plans with those whom you advise about their careers.

Consider the extent to which you (i) have the knowledge and skills and (ii) practise them – in your relationships with those you advise about their career and in your everyday working life in other aspects of your job (you might generalise the items in the list above to 'colleague or member of staff'). Complete your audit checklist in Table 8.2 as you did for Table 8.1, considering how expert you are (*see* page 45).

Table 8.2:   Self-check of own knowledge and skills in respect of personal and people development

Aspect of personal and people development	How expert are you? Aware? Competent? Expert?	How frequently do you use these? At least: every day? Weekly? Monthly?
Understanding healthcare context relevant to you and others		
Understanding healthcare priorities		
Evaluating own knowledge and practice		
Applying own learning arising from PDP		
Recognising what others have learnt and achieved		
Working with others in relation to careers advice to implement learning		
Negotiating goal setting, action planning etc		

Understanding the healthcare context and priorities

You need to be familiar with the main NHS strategies driving developments nationally, and local opportunities. Find out more about any professional requirements of individuals you advise about their careers from the relevant Royal Colleges or other professional bodies. Keep up to date with changes in postgraduate education and career progression.

Force-field analysis[10]

Use a force-field analysis exercise with the person you are informing or advising to try to identify any significant source of unhappiness for the person in relation to their career. Just as in medicine, if the diagnosis is wrong the treatment won't work. It is essential to be clear about exactly what is causing the unhappiness and make sure it is indeed their career itself. It won't help them to uproot everything and change jobs only to find they have taken the same problems with them.

Using a force-field analysis approach helps people to identify and focus down on the positive and negative forces in their work and/or home lives, and to gain an overview of the relative weighting of these factors. The exercise is suitable for anyone and everyone at any stage in their career. You can use it to show them how to review their own circumstances and need for career development.

The student or doctor you are advising about their career should draw a horizontal or vertical line in the middle of a sheet of paper. One side should be 'positive' and the other side 'negative'. They should then draw arrows to represent individual positive drivers that motivate them on one side of the line, and negative factors that demotivate them on the other negative side of the line. The chunkiness and length of the arrows should represent the extent of the influence; that is, a short, narrow arrow will indicate that the positive or negative factor has a minor influence, and a long, wide arrow a major effect.

The analysis helps people to realise whether a known influence in their life is a positive or negative factor. For instance they may realise upon reflection that they had assumed that money in the form of a good salary was a positive motivator. But really, the wish to sustain or increase their income was a negative force on their job satisfaction, due to their inability to spend time on meaningful non-pecuniary work-related activities.

The next step is for them to make a personal or organisational action plan to create the situations and opportunities to boost the positive factors in their life and minimise arrows on the negative side. They could invite someone who knows them well to review the force-field analysis they have drawn and let them know honestly of any blind-spots and if they have the positive and negative influences in proportion. Then they can determine their needs and priorities that should be addressed in planning for the change. This can be done through:

- changing the strength of a driving force: width and length of the arrows
- changing the direction of a force: switching a force to be positive rather than restraining
- withdrawing or minimising a restraining force
- adding or enlarging helping, positive forces (*see* Figure 8.5).

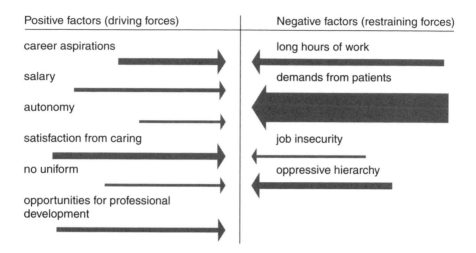

Figure 8.5: Example of a force-field analysis diagram: satisfaction with current post as a doctor.

Bridging the gap[12]

Help the student or doctor you are advising to confront the gap between 'where they want to be' and 'where they are now'. This gap then becomes central to a planned programme of personal development and change, the nature of which depends on the various gaps identified and their future goals. Visualise their progress using Figure 8.6.

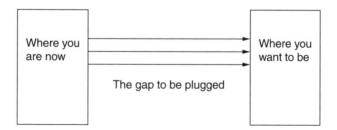

Figure 8.6:   An outline gap analysis.

This exercise is hard and requires a certain amount of insight from the person you are advising. You can help guide them even better if you have done your own gap analysis as preparation for your own careers adviser role (*see* Box 8.4).

Box 8.4:   Work out your own gap analysis

1   *Where you are now*: this will include a description of the important aspects of your work/home situation that are relevant to the goals you envisage and changes you want to make. It may cover your strengths and weaknesses in your current role, your experience, your transferable skills, a review of how your current post measures up to your expectations and values. It might also include a SWOT analysis of your strengths, weaknesses, opportunities and threats (*see* page 96).

2   *Define your future goals*: be as specific as you can be about what you want to achieve. Describe your interests, areas of work and development you'd like to be responsible for or involved in, setting you wish to work in, or type of role. Outline your aspirations and preferences. At this stage you can be as inventive or imaginative as you want to be. What would an ideal world look like?

3   *Describe the gap*: compare items 1 and 2 and describe the main differences between your current state and your desired future position. Make a plan for change with timescales and milestones so that you can monitor progress. Discuss your plan with others who know you, for a reality check. Outline the opportunities that might link where you are now with your future goals.

Change[10]

There are lots of reasons why colleagues may be hesitant about changing the way they do things. The barriers to making and sustaining change are many and varied. People sometimes underestimate the hurdles to be overcome before change can be made, and are therefore sometimes surprised at how difficult it can become.[13] Some of these barriers are listed below:

- lack of perception of relevance of proposed change (is it your idea or the person whom you are advising?)
- lack of resources to make change happen
- short-term outlook
- conflicting priorities
- lack of necessary skills
- limited evidence of effectiveness of proposed change
- perverse incentives (are there factors that make it more attractive to stay put?)
- the intensity of personal contribution required
- having a poor appreciation of the need to change, or considering the need to change to be secondary to other issues
- having a poor understanding of the proposed solutions, or considering the solution to be inappropriate
- disagreeing about how the change should be implemented
- embarrassment about admitting that what you are doing could be improved.

Change will not be possible unless those you are advising have thought through their career plan thoroughly, are committed to it and prepared to alter factors in their lives so that it is possible to make the change happen in practice.

You need to help others to face up to change by identifying the causes for dis-satisfaction with the present situation, to have a clear idea of where they are heading. They should map out how to reach their targets, then find their way in staged steps to measure the progress towards the target.

Tips for making changes

It might help to give those you advise a checklist for planning change that they can adapt to their particular situation:

- have realistic time scales and be flexible
- provide clear communication about what is happening
- consult with all the staff, identifying all the problems as they occur
- plan for more resources and time than you expect to use
- fix interval markers of progress
- feed the information back to people about what is happening
- identify the anxieties and try to resolve them
- consider the effects of this change on other services and people
- beware of too many changes taking place at once
- recognise that change can be hijacked by vested interests and the direction altered
- be prepared to change direction if necessary
- beware of a lack of commitment from others.

Understanding the influence of people's personality type

Understanding more about their personality type can help people to make a rational choice about the type of career track they should follow. Career and personality match are very important – as are their personal preferences for their balance between work and leisure, work and income, degree of responsibility, type of work, and extent of interaction with people.

Knowing more about yourself, your personality and emotions, will help you to interact with and manage other people better. Feelings are highly influenced by your personality and your value system, all part of emotional intelligence.

Personality profile tests attempt to show individuals their preferred style of behav-iour, in order that they can then choose the aspect of their profession that best matches the way they behave. Opinions about the benefits of psychometric testing are divided. The aim of the test is to identify a person's preferred way of behaving, based on their individual ways of perceiving the world and exercising judgement, in order to help in every aspect of life, career and personal relationships.

There are many varieties of personality profile questionnaires. Three of the best known are the Myers Briggs type indicator, the Sci45, and the 16PF questionnaire which assesses 16 personality factors.[14,15]

The Sci45 is a validated psychometric instrument designed by the Open University for selection of medical specialties by doctors in training.[14] It provides career guidance based on the fit between the skill, aspiration, personal preference and attribute profile of the trainee, and the characteristics of available training specialties. The Sci45 is thought to be most appropriate for trainees who are unsure of what medical career path to follow (*see* Chapter 2).

The Myers Briggs profile has four dimensions:[15]

- *E or I; extroversion or introversion*: how you focus your attention, either in the outside world (extroversion) or in your head (introversion)
- *S or N; sensing or intuition*: the way you prefer to take in and process information, either literally (sensing) or generally and in patterns (intuition)
- *T or F; thinking or feeling*: how you make decisions, either logical and objective (thinking) or value based and people oriented (feeling)
- *J or P; judging or perceiving*: whether you live in a scheduled and organised way (judging) or are spontaneous and flexible (perceiving).

There is no right or wrong personality, just different personalities that work more or less effectively depending on the situation people are in. There is no ideal personality fit for a particular job, and a mix of different personalities within the same specialty or workforce group brings fresh perspectives and balance to the work team. For many people, becoming more aware of their personal preferences and styles means that they gain confidence and pride in their own characteristics, rather than seeking to conform to an imagined stereotype.

Helping others to understand themselves better will help them to realise their potential. The shy, inward looking person is not going to enjoy a work situation that calls for constant interaction, and the gregarious extrovert will become depressed if they are deprived of social contact. Understanding their own personal preferences and nature and what they want out of life should help them to embark on or develop an appropriate career path (*see* Box 8.5).

Box 8.5:   About personality type

- There is no right or wrong, better or worse combinations of personality types.
- If you know more about your type you can understand yourself better.
- Each person is unique.
- Everyone uses each of their preferences to some degree.
- The human personality is too complex for type to explain everything about you.

Find out which facilitators or consultants can provide an analysis of a personality profile in your locality. Ask the education or learning lead in your deanery or trust for contact details, or look for possibilities on the web. Warn the doctors you are advising that they may have to pay for a resource such as this in a private capacity.

Assist in maintaining others' health, safety and security

Promote others' health, safety and security by:

- being familiar with resources to which you can signpost a person you are advising about their career, for help or advice e.g. occupational health, stress, financial or relationship difficulties, both within and outside the NHS
- helping those you advise to identify risks in relation to their health, safety and security

- being clear what constitutes careers advice or guidance and what is outside your scope in respect of health or counselling issues
- understanding and reporting any issues or serious concerns that could affect patient care with explicit consent of those you advise; without consent if patient safety seems to be at risk.

Consider the extent to which you (i) have the knowledge and skills and (ii) practise them – in your relationship with individuals whom you advise about their careers and in your everyday working life in other aspects of your job (you might generalise the items in the list above to 'colleague or member of staff'). Complete your audit checklist in Table 8.3 as you did for Table 8.1, considering how expert you are (*see* page 45).

Table 8.3:   Self-check of your own knowledge and skills in respect of maintaining health, safety and security

Aspect of health, safety and security	How expert are you? Aware? Competent? Expert?	How frequently do you use these? At least: every day? weekly? monthly?
Being familiar with network to signpost others for help		
Helping others identify risks in relation to health, safety, security		
Being clear what constitutes careers information, advice or guidance, and the boundaries		
Understanding and reporting issues that put patient safety at risk		

Signposting individuals to other resources as part of a career discussion

If you are to sustain your role as careers adviser or guide without moving into other roles such as counsellor, mentor or providing pastoral support, you need to be familiar with what local resources there are within and outside the NHS, and know how others may access them. Compile a logbook of resources, access arrangements and contact details and local protocols covering the following:

- occupational health support: for ill and distressed individuals, those with alcohol or drug misuse problems, those whose physical or mental disabilities create functional problems
- local process for poor or underperformance of the person you are advising, or for them to use if they are concerned about their colleagues
- stress management help

- explicit protocols for informing others if you suspect that patient safety is at risk according to whether those whom you advise do, or do not, continue to work
- processes and resources for signposting educational support for general or specific learning and development needs that are, or are not, recognised by those you advise
- resources for career development: what is available and contact details
- advice on financial difficulties
- counselling for relationship difficulties, within and outside the work setting
- careers information about access to a wide range of medically related careers
- career counselling
- guarantee of indemnity for you as a careers adviser in the unlikely event that an individual you have advised makes an official complaint: information about explicit limits of indemnity
- trouble-shooting guide: someone or sources of help to consult if problems arise – relating to any/all of above.

Minimise stress[16]

Stress can be either positive or negative, depending on how you perceive it and how you react to it. If individuals you advise view sources of stress such as new regulations, as challenges rather than burdens, they will probably find ways of managing changes to their advantage with opportunities for learning and growth.

Symptoms of poor fit between their personality type and the job might include feeling:

- tired, stressed or depressed
- incompetent
- unvalued
- misunderstood
- unable to use their strengths.

The common sources of stress described in Box 8.6 are those that people with different personality profiles (categorised by Myers Briggs[15]) are prone to. The more you can help those who consult you about their careers to understand personality-related reasons for any current dissatisfaction with their jobs, the less likely they are to make unnecessary changes of job, but instead work on resolving current conflicts.

Box 8.6:   Common sources of stress for different character types[16,17]

- *Extroverts*: too much time alone, solitary tasks.
- *Introverts*: too many new people, not enough time alone.
- *Intuitives*: too many details, lack of autonomy.
- *Sensors*: uncertainty, lack of clarity, too much change, complexity, need to make long-term plans.
- *Thinkers*: emotional situations, disregard of logic, poor results from careful planning, hurting others' feelings while in pursuit of goals.
- *Feelers*: conflict, giving too much, violation of core values, perception that a problem is their fault, hurting someone despite best intentions.
- *Judgers*: unexpected events disrupting careful plans, disorganisation, overwork.
- *Perceivers*: tight deadlines or too much structure, situations where all options are closed.

Unchecked, any or all of these sources of stress may eventually lead to performance problems at work and/or ill-health. The more that a person understands how important it is that their personality type is matched with the nature of their day-to-day work, the more this will help them to get the right balance between contact with people or patients, and thinking or managing.

Promote job satisfaction and career fulfilment

Job satisfaction is known to protect people from the effects of stress from work. So increasing job satisfaction is one of the best ways you can recommend someone 'stress proofs' themselves against the pressures and demands of a job. They will minimise the effects of the elements of the job they find more stressful if they enjoy their job, feel valued and are in control of their everyday work.[18,19]

Stress management[20]

In general stress management should include three approaches:

1 *Thinking*
For example:

- think more positively
- put things in perspective and think longer-term
- be more flexible
- find ways to control your thinking style.

2 *Behaviour*
For example:

- talk about your worries to those at work who are responsible for the stress or are in a position to alleviate it
- seek support from friends and family
- be proactive about controlling stress-provoking factors
- be assertive
- manage your time effectively.

3 *Health*
For example:

- achieve a better work/life balance
- find methods of relaxation that work for you
- follow a healthy lifestyle.

Contribute to service improvement and quality improvement (through effective careers information/advice)

Contribute to the development of careers advice services for students and doctors by:

- encouraging reflective practice to enable those you are advising to learn from their own experiences

- demonstrating personal commitment to quality improvement in general
- offering advice and support in relation to quality improvement in career advisory services
- monitoring your own performance as a careers adviser or guide and taking action to improve your performance in this role
- maintaining knowledge and information resources relating to medical careers
- helping others to access and use information and resources relating to medical careers.

Consider the extent to which you (i) have the knowledge and skills, and (ii) practise them – in your relationship with those you appraise and in your everyday working life in other aspects of your job (you might generalise the items in the list above to 'colleague or member of staff'). Complete your audit checklist below in Table 8.4 as you did for Table 8.1, considering how expert you are (*see* page 45).

Table 8.4: Self-check of own knowledge and skills in respect of service improvement and quality improvement

Aspect of service development	How expert are you? Aware? Competent? Expert?	How frequently do you use these? At least: every day? weekly? monthly?
Encouraging others in reflective practice		
Demonstrating personal commitment to quality improvement in general		
Offering advice in improving careers advisory services		
Monitoring own performance as careers adviser		
Maintaining knowledge and information resources relating to medical careers		
Helping others to access and use information and resources relating to medical careers		

Reflective practice

Knowles has defined seven fundamentals as guidelines to encourage adult learners in reflective practice, which are relevant to those being appraised:[21]

1 establish an effective learning climate where people feel safe and comfortable expressing themselves
2 involve individuals in mutual planning of relevant methods and curricular content

3 trigger internal motivation by involving individuals in diagnosing their own needs
4 give others more control by encouraging them to formulate their own learning objectives
5 encourage those you are appraising to identify resources and devise strategies for using the resources to achieve their objectives
6 support others in carrying out their learning plans
7 develop individuals' skills of critical reflection by involving them in evaluating their own learning.

Learning should be a continuous process of investigation, exploration, action, reflection and further action.

Strengths, weaknesses, opportunities and threats (SWOT) analysis during the careers discussion: help others to identify priorities for service development and improve services[10]

This classic strategic planning technique can be used by those you advise to analyse their internal capability, and to set that in relation to service development relating to work.

They should undertake a SWOT analysis of their own performance with you, on their own, or with a group of colleagues. Brainstorm the strengths, weaknesses (or challenges), opportunities and threats of their situation using Box 8.7 as a template.

Strengths and weaknesses of individuals might include: knowledge, experience, expertise, decision making, communication, interprofessional relationships, political skills, time keeping, organisation, teaching and research. Strengths and weaknesses for the organisation might relate to most of these aspects too, as well as resources – staff, skills or structural items.

Opportunities might relate to unexploited potential strengths, expected changes, options for career development pathways, hobbies and interests that could usefully be expanded.

Threats will include factors and circumstances that prevent them from achieving their aims for personal, professional and team development, and improvements in patient care.

The SWOT analysis creates opportunities to learn, at the same time as undertaking the actual needs analysis.

Box 8.7:   SWOT analysis: how to do it

The person undertaking the SWOT analysis should write on a single flip chart/ sheet of paper so that they can see all four quadrants at once.

Strengths	Weaknesses
Opportunities	Threats

Each section is then completed. For example:

1 *strengths*: what am I good at? What factors are in my favour?
2 *weaknesses*: what am I not so good at?
3 *opportunities*: what's likely to be useful that I could harness? What is happening that could help me? What is new, and is it good for me?
4 *threats*: what could be a threat to my/our achievements? What's new and is it bad for me?

Prioritise important factors. Draw up goals and a timed action plan.

Now they should compare what they have produced with what a colleague thought when they addressed the same task. Discuss any differences with them. Describe what they need to learn more about to address the goals they have set for their career path or their knowledge and skills.

By the end of the SWOT analysis they should be at the stage where they can move on to considering:

- how can I optimise and extend the strengths identified?
- how can I minimise or overcome the weaknesses?
- how can I make most use of the opportunities?
- how can I avoid the threats or counter their effects?

Significant event analysis[22]

Significant event audit is a structured approach to helping the student or doctor you are advising review events that have occurred at work or in their career so far. Such events might be in any area of their career: failing to get an interview, being unsuccessful at interview, receiving a poor reference, work-related stress. Look back at the list of career crises given on pages 59–60 – any of these might warrant a significant event audit. Significant event auditing should be a positive developmental process.

   The doctor concerned should discuss the significant event at a designated meeting with colleagues in their team, family members or whoever is relevant to the event.

Track through the circumstances and all factors relating to the event from everyone's perspectives, respecting their insights. Determine what lessons can be learned, what areas require further work on your part, how things can be improved, who is responsible for the action plan and by when.

Demonstrating your competence as a careers adviser or guide to medical students and/or doctors[23]

See Chapter 9 for more information on this approach.

Knowledge and information resources

The scope of this area and sources of information were well covered in Chapter 3. Look out for search tools like *JobScore* (*see* page 25).

Support equality and value diversity

Support people's equality and value diversity by:

- being aware of *your own* values, beliefs and attitudes and seeking to use these in a constructive manner in the interests of those you advise
- making evaluations and providing feedback that is free of bias and prejudice; being open and transparent in dealings involving those you inform or advise
- having a cultural awareness
- demonstrating personal commitment to equality and diversity.

Consider the extent to which you (i) have the knowledge and skills and (ii) practise them – in your relationship with individuals you advise and in your everyday working life in other aspects of your job (you might generalise the items in the list above to 'colleague or member of staff'). Complete your audit checklist in Table 8.5 as you did for Table 8.1 considering how expert you are (*see* page 45).

Table 8.5: Self-check of own knowledge and skills in respect of supporting equality and valuing diversity in relation to careers information and advice

Aspect of service development	How expert are you? Aware? Competent? Expert?	How frequently do you use these? At least: every day? weekly? monthly?
Using awareness of *own* values, beliefs and attitudes in constructive manner		
Making evaluations and providing feedback free of bias and prejudice; being open and transparent		
Having cultural awareness		
Demonstrating personal commitment to equality and diversity		

Know what equality means and who may be affected

Equality is about everyone being able to participate and have the opportunity to fulfil their potential. It is backed by legislation designed to address unfair discrimination based on membership of a particular group. Such groups include black and minority ethnic people, disabled people, women, gay, lesbian, transgender and bisexual people – that may be under-represented in specific parts of the workforce. It also includes those who feel they have been, or may be, discriminated against or disadvantaged due to factors such as social background, age or religion.[24]

Equality and diversity are not interchangeable. They need to be progressed together. There is no equality of opportunity if difference is not recognised and valued. Diversity is about the recognition and valuing of difference in its broadest sense. It is about creating a working culture and practices that recognise, respect, value and harness difference for the benefit of the NHS and the individual, including patients.[24]

The principle of equal opportunity should apply to employment, training, education, provision of goods, facilities or services. The principle of equal treatment guarantees freedom of discrimination on the grounds of sex, pregnancy, marital status, family status and gender reassignment.[25]

Know the meaning of diversity and why it is important to value it

Value diversity – for it is the contrast and differences in views, style, attitudes, ethnic origins, life experiences and personality between people that provides energy and ideas. Exposing elements of diversity can be potentially threatening, as people fear that elements of themselves they would rather keep secret may be exposed (look back at the thinking around the façade and blind area in the JoHari window model on pages 79–81). So be sensitive to diversity.

Giving effective feedback

Look back at page 83 to remind yourself of the principles and practice of giving constructive and fair feedback that is free of bias and prejudice.

Review case histories of doctors who have overcome illness, disability or prejudice

Be inspired, impressed and enlightened by reading and reflecting on the experiences of doctors and medical students who have faced up to illness, disability and discrimination. Read up about them, and recommend others to do the same.[26]

References

1 Department of Health (2004) *The NHS Knowledge and Skills Framework (NHS KSF) and Development Review Guidance*. Version 7. London: Department of Health, London.

2 Department of Health (2003) *Agenda for Change. Proposed agreement*. Department of Health, London.

3 Eraut M and du Boulay B (2002) *Developing the Attributes of Medical Professional Judgement and Competence*. University of Sussex, Sussex. www.informatics.sussex.ac.uk/users/bend/doh (accessed 10 August 2005).

4 Bhargie ODW (1997) *The Handbook of Communication Skills* (2e). Routledge, London.

5 Tate P (2000) *The Doctors' Communication Handbook* (3e). Radcliffe Medical Press, London.

6 Benner P (1984) *From Novice to Expert*. Addison-Wesley, London.

7 Alder H (1996) *NLP for Managers. How to achieve excellence at work*. Piatkus, London.

8 Luft J (1970) *Group Processes: an introduction to group dynamics* (2e). National Press Books, Palo Alto, California.

9 Scholtes P (1998) *The Leader's Handbook, Making Things Happen Getting Things Done*. McGraw Hill, Maidenhead.

10 Chambers R, Wakley G, Iqbal Z and Field S (2002) *Prescription for Learning. Techniques, games and activities*. Radcliffe Medical Press, Oxford.

11 Mohanna K, Wall D and Chambers R (2004) *Teaching Made Easy. A manual for health professionals* (2e). Radcliffe Medical Press, Oxford.

12 Bayley H, Donovan C and Chambers R (2004) *Good Mentoring Toolkit*. Radcliffe Medical Press, Oxford.

13 Elwyn G, Greenhalgh T, MacFarlane F and Koppel S (2001) *Groups – a guide to small group work in healthcare, management, education and research*. Radcliffe Medical Press, Oxford.

14 Gale R and Grant J (2002) Sci45: the development of a specialty choice inventory. *Medical Education*. **36:** 659–66.

15 Briggs Myers I and Myers P (1995) *Gifts Differing. Understanding personality type*. Davies-Black Publishing, Palo Alto, California.

16 Chambers R (1998) *Survival Skills for GPs*. Radcliffe Medical Press, Oxford.

17 Houghton A (2005) What do type dynamics tell us about life stages and stress reactions? *BMJ Careers*. **1 January:** 8–9.

18 Sutherland V and Cooper C (1993) Identifying distress among general practitioners: predictors of psychological ill-health and job dissatisfaction. *Social Science and Medicine*. **37:** 575–81.

19 Ramirez A, Graham J, Richards M *et al.* (1996) Mental health of hospital consultants: the effects of stress and satisfaction at work. *The Lancet*. **347:** 724–8.

20 Chambers R, Schwartz A and Boath E (2003) *Beating Stress in the NHS*. Radcliffe Medical Press, Oxford.

21 Knowles MS (1984) *Andragogy in Action: applying modern principles of adult learning*. Jossey-Bass, San Francisco.

22 Chambers R and Wakley G (2005) *Clinical Audit in Primary Care: quality and outcomes*. Radcliffe Publishing, Oxford.

23 Chambers R, Mohanna K, Wakley G and Wall D (2004) *Demonstrating Your Competence 1. Healthcare teaching*. Radcliffe Medical Press, Oxford.

24 Department of Health (2004) *Sharing the Challenge, Sharing the Benefits – equality and diversity in the medical workforce*. Department of Health, London.

25 Equal Opportunities Commission (1998) *Equality in the 21st Century*. Equal Opportunities Commission, Manchester.

26 MacDonald R (2004) Training and Working with Disabilities. Career focus information guide. *BMJ Careers supplement*.

9

Demonstrating your competence as a careers adviser

Ruth Chambers

As a professional, you should be able to demonstrate your competence in the roles of your daily work – for appraisal or revalidation of your professional qualifications. If you are providing careers information or advice you should gather evidence that you are staying up to date and maintaining your competence in the careers field as well as in other areas of your work.

Box 9.1 summarises a description of an effective careers adviser – but how can you demonstrate this or show that you are working towards deserving this description?

Box 9.1: Summary: being effective in providing careers information and/or advice to medical students or doctors

Here is a checklist for you. Do you:

- put your main effort into trying to understand the other person? Every person is unique – respect the other person's view of the world
- develop a range of styles for working with others? Do not just rely on one or two ways
- ask open questions and show you are using active listening skills?
- create a real rapport with appropriate non-verbal communication?
- ask for feedback? Are you aware of yourself and how you appear to others?
- understand that every behaviour is useful in some way, and use this knowledge?

The stages of the evidence cycle for demonstrating your standards of practice or competence and any necessary improvements in your practice as a mentor are given in Figure 9.1. Although the five stages are shown in sequence here, in practice you would expect to move backwards and forwards from stage to stage, because of new information or a modification of your earlier ideas. New information might accrue which affects your approach to providing careers advice. A critical incident or complaint from someone you advised might occur which causes you and others to think anew about the way you work. The arrows in Figure 9.1 show that you might reset your target or aspirations for good practice having undertaken exercises to identify what you need to learn, or determine whether there are deficiencies in the way you provide careers information or advice.

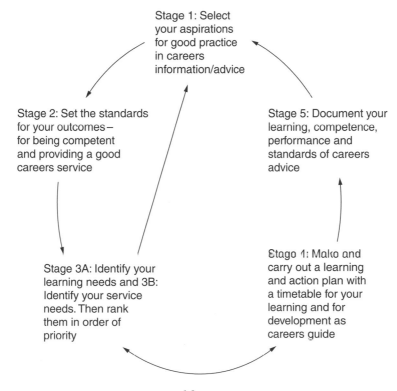

Figure 9.1: Stages of the evidence cycle.[1,2]

As you start to collate information around this five-stage cycle, discuss any problems about providing careers information and/or advice with colleagues, experts in this area, tutors, etc. You will want to develop a wide range and depth of evidence so that you can show that you are competent in your day-to-day general work as well as your expertise in providing careers support.

You should be able to demonstrate that you can maintain a satisfactory standard most of the time in how you provide careers information or advice, and in your everyday work. Some of the time you will be brilliant, of course! Celebrate those moments. On other occasions, you or others will be critical of your performance and feel that you could have done much better or identified the need for additional resources. Reflect on those episodes to learn from them.

Illustrative example of evidence to demonstrate that you are competent at providing careers information and/or advice

The following example gives an illustrative cycle of evidence you might use or adapt to enable you to gather evidence that you are performing well.[2] You might want to copy the example in your own practice, or adapt it and draw up your own approach to gathering evidence to show that you are competent in providing careers support.

Case study: Providing careers information and careers advice

Robert has just finished his second post in his Foundation 2 year. He is consulting you as you walk into the postgraduate centre together as he knows you have given careers advice to some of his colleagues. He wonders what you think of his plans to travel round the world before settling down into a hospital-based career, probably in a medical specialty. Will he be able to get a job on his return? Will travelling spoil his chances of a good medical career? What are his chances of making it as a consultant in a specialty like respiratory medicine? He is suddenly free to travel after the break up of his long-term relationship with his girlfriend.

Stage 1: Select your aspirations for good practice

The excellent careers adviser:

- establishes an honest and trustworthy relationship with the person they are advising
- guides the person for whom they are providing careers information and advice to take up appropriate personal, professional and career development opportunities.

Stage 2: Set the standards for your outcomes

Outcomes might include:

- the way learning or good practice is applied
- a learnt skill
- a protocol
- meeting recommended standards.

- Establish a good and open relationship between both parties, by adopting formative and supportive roles.
- The person you are advising about their career gains new insights and perspectives and enjoys being challenged to develop their career.

Stage 3A: Identify your learning needs

If you have not started to provide careers information and/or advice yet and are considering doing so:

- reflect on the good qualities of a doctor who provides careers information and/or advice and check the extent to which you already have those qualities by discussion with a trusted colleague or friend. Ask them if they would provide a fictional reference for you for a potential medical student or doctor seeking your careers advice, as an exercise for you to read and consider their perspectives
- talk to doctors and others (e.g. personnel staff) who provide careers advice to medical students or doctors: what is their time commitment, how do they deal with interpersonal conflicts, do they provide follow-up advice sessions? Compare with your capacity and approach for providing careers support in your current role and your degree of commitment
- in your discussion with the deanery lead for careers support for doctors, find out how much training is provided or available, and what ongoing support is arranged
- obtain a job description for the role of careers adviser, or ask the deanery lead to write one if none exists; make a judgement of whether you have sufficient knowledge and skills or training needs.

If you do provide careers information and/or advice already:

- work out a system to ask the last three students or doctors whom you have advised or helped with careers information for their honest appraisal of your strengths and weaknesses in your role
- participate in role-play exercises at training and support sessions using case studies, and receive peer feedback on your attitudes and responses.

Stage 3B: Identify your service needs

> Any of the needs assessment exercises in 3A may also reveal service needs.

- Ask the deanery lead for provision of careers support to doctors for anonymised feedback from the people for whom you have provided help.

Stage 4: Make and carry out a learning and action plan

- Attend a training workshop for new or potential careers advisers for medical students and/or doctors. Discuss how to help a young doctor in Robert's situation and cope with the other factors going on in young doctors' lives that impact on their career choices.
- Talk to doctors or other personnel who provide such careers information and advice. Find out what it is they most value about the role and their top tips and techniques. Learn from those with experience how to maintain limits to careers guidance discussions, and signpost on those students or doctors needing help for other factors such as ill-health, stress, financial concerns.

- Learn how to record and use informal feedback by discussion with others at peer group meetings.
- Find out about sources of reference for reliable careers information that you can share with those whom you are helping. Also learn what practical support is available in your locality or from professional organisations to allow study leave, shadowing, secondments etc.

Stage 5: Document your learning, competence, performance and standards of careers advice

- Keep a job description for your role, with written reflections as to your knowledge and skills and training needs and how they will or have been met.
- Keep a record of feedback from a person or people for whom you have provided careers information and/or advice – or from role-plays at a workshop. Note your reflections on this feedback.
- Make notes of key points and contact details, from what you have learnt from reading and reference material.

Case study continued

You book an appointment to talk to Robert later in the week. The initial training you undertook at a careers workshop and follow-up session pays off as you already have lots of material to hand about qualifications, competition ratios in specialties he is interested in, and practical help, that is useful to Rob in making his career choices. He particularly benefits from your skills at challenging his perceptions and perspectives and goes on to complete his Foundation Year 2 posts, taking exciting holidays rather than a career break.

References

1 Chambers R, Wakley G, Field S and Ellis S (2003) *Appraisal for the Apprehensive.* Radcliffe Medical Press, Oxford.

2 Chambers R, Mohanna K, Wakley G and Wall D (2004) *Demonstrating Your Competence 1: healthcare teaching.* Radcliffe Medical Press, Oxford.

10

Establishing a careers strategy

Ruth Chambers

This chapter contains material you could adapt for drawing up a strategy in your locality – your deanery, your health authority area, your trust or organisation. It has been derived from workshops and preliminary work in evolving a careers strategy for the West Midlands deanery. Any careers strategy should be based on the components recommended by the *Modernising Medical Careers* Working Group for career management for doctors (*see* Chapter 2).[1]

Establish your vision

How about the following:

All medical students and doctors working and training in the XXX region or contemplating a return to practice or move to the region, can access well-informed careers information, guidance and counselling when they require it.

You might wish to extend your vision to include dentists or other healthcare professionals.

Specify the principles on which your strategy is based

For instance:

- every doctor should be on a career pathway during the whole of their careers – not just at the beginning
- career decision making is a lifetime continuum, with a focus in the early years of a doctor's career
- all doctors should be linked to some sort of training, and their development needs should be assessed by regular appraisal
- the career support needs of some target groups have a higher priority than others (e.g. Foundation Year 2 doctors make significant career choices early in their careers)

- careers support services are an essential feature of the training and development a doctor should expect from the deanery or trust employing them
- the deanery should enable individual doctors, SHAs and employing trusts, to realise the benefits of accessible and available careers support services. This includes enabling individuals to utilise careers information, advice and guidance to gain insights into the careers for which they are suited, and range of careers opportunities
- careers support services should support career choices and the needs of the individual doctor should be balanced against the demands of the service in an open and transparent way
- careers support services should cater for all individuals whatever their circumstances, and be able to handle complex situations including doctors about whom there are concerns or who have personal difficulties
- educators and others providing careers support to doctors should have the dedicated time and competence to do so.

Target groups – to whom your strategy relates

These might include:

- school children and non-medical graduates with potential to become medical students (all backgrounds)
- medical students
- Foundation Year l doctors
- Foundation Year 2 doctors
- other junior doctors including specialist registrars
- non-consultant career grade doctors
- established GPs
- specialist doctors employed by the NHS
- specialist doctors working outside the NHS
- doctors with potential to return to practice
- doctors who qualified overseas (in an EU or in non-EU country, refugee doctors)
- NHS managers/workforce planners.

Relevant factors or characteristics of your target groups for whom you may need to make special provision include:

- seniority
- specialty
- skills
- age
- sex
- disability (new; long-term/short-term; congenital)
- country of training and qualification
- competition ratios.

Potential provision

Consider what information, advice, guidance and counselling sources you want to include and who will provide them. Select from the lists below and specify who will provide what, when, where, how etc.

- *Careers information*:
  - deanery and trust websites
  - HR/personnel/line managers
- *Careers advice and guidance*:
  - peers (trained peer careers advisers will also become careers advice enthusiasts)
  - educational supervisors
  - clinical tutors
  - college tutors
  - appraisers (appraisers of Foundation Years 1 and 2 doctors must include 'career plan review')
  - mentors
  - deanery and trust staff (administration)
  - specialty recruiters
  - postgraduate medical library staff
  - professional bodies
  - Royal Colleges and their representatives
- *Career counselling*:
  - career counsellors.

Components of the vision

The infrastructure required to provide all doctors working in the deanery/trust/ organisation or contemplating a return to practice with access to well informed careers information, guidance and counselling includes the following headings.

Careers information should be readily available and promoted in a timely manner

Accessible careers information which should give information on:

- the range of jobs available
- qualifications/training required
- regulations
- personal perspectives
- local and national competition ratios
- local information: schools, jobs centres (for other family members) – people need access to early information at school level.

This might be available as a gateway via the deanery/trust website to be linked to SHAs', trusts', Royal Colleges' websites. Careers information should be individualised for particular groups of doctors: for instance, Foundation Year doctors, refugee and overseas-trained doctors.

Regular open days or careers fairs could be run by the deanery for people contemplating a career in medicine, and for established doctors and dentists or those in training. All such groups should participate in hosting the careers fairs to share their experiences. The way careers fairs are run should be reviewed to assess their effectiveness, and organisers should describe their purpose, and plan how they might be improved to meet visitors' needs.

All doctors should have a PDP which is relevant to their career path. Illustrative career pathways should be published. A nominated member of staff in the deanery or trust should keep a watching brief to update the published careers information, including changes to contact details, competition ratios etc.

A careers advisory service should:

- provide impartial advice or guidance on career choices
- provide informed guidance on an individual's suitability for specific medical careers
- be available at set times within the training and qualifications structure
- provide (i) clinical guidance and (ii) HR guidance (e.g. for CV, interview skills) at local level
- be offered to all doctors in training
- be available to doctors at all stages of their career
- include mentors for doctors with specific career needs
- include mentors or role models for career specialties which are less popular or have most vacancies (e.g. academic career)
- have a flexible ethos, to enable doctors to recognise the uncertain nature of their future career in a continually changing NHS.

There should be a database and directory of those with dedicated time who are recognised as competent to give careers advice and guidance, to provide choice for doctors wishing to access such help, or for their educational supervisors to direct trainees towards help.

Competent careers advisers/guides will be able to help trainees who are not suited to a career specialty, or do not have the aptitude for a chosen career path, to gain insight into the mismatch between their aspirations and reality (this may require access to personality profile testing to increase insight into their own strengths and preferences with feedback/discussion from the adviser).

Careers advice should be individualised for those considering a return to practice.

A career counselling service should be available to doctors when careers guidance has proved insufficient for their needs

Access should be with the support of person providing careers guidance. Career counselling service should offer (in rank order):

- remedial action for underperformance
- generic career counselling as option- not specialty-specific
- sources of appropriate support

- facilitation of individual doctors at times of 'crisis'
- personality profiling: for doctors with attitudinal and interpersonal problems
- a service that can 'match' a person with career specialism or mode of working; helping them face up to their lack of suitability for a particular specialism
- an ability to provide help and support for trauma of career counselling – and coming to terms with limited career choices or unwanted insights.

Career counselling should enable the person to come to an informed and rational decision about where to go next. It should enable people to reflect on, and appreciate, their own strengths and weaknesses.

Enabling career planning and management

Established doctors and those in training should be enabled to take an active part in planning their own career pathways via access to careers information (paper and electronic), career management workshops, software to help with decision support in careers, and careers advisory services, for example, a session on careers management as part of the Foundation Year 2 teaching programme. The ethos would be to help trainees take responsibility for their own careers.

Access to supported personality profile testing, e.g. Sci45 CD profile and feedback should be possible.

Competence of those providing careers information, advice or guidance to doctors

All educators and deanery staff should be able to signpost doctors and others in the target group of this strategy to reliable careers information. A proportion will be trained and competent as careers advisers. A few will be trained and competent as career counsellors (perhaps two or three trained consultants and a nominated member of HR covering one or a group of hospitals).

The deanery should arrange initial training and updates so that those providing careers information, or advice and guidance are:

- well informed
- empathic with individual doctors and dentists or other clients
- obvious at local level (CPD tutors, course organisers, university staff, deanery staff, health librarians, trust staff, appraisers, College representatives)
- competent with demonstrable knowledge and skills in equity and diversity
- able to signpost doctors or dentists to reliable and useful sources of information
- at least competent
- able to engage with people
- aware of their limitations
- able to refer doctor to expert career resources
- able to access to careers support resources.

The deanery should develop networks of role models who have achieved senior positions in medical specialties who are willing to share their experience and guide others in relation to accessing the career path, especially in shortage specialties (but those involved in this initiative should have a good mix of people prepared to be nominated as role models to guard against stereotyping certain roles).

All educational supervisors and clinical tutors should have a positive attitude and minimum levels of career guidance knowledge and skills. Others (such as CPD tutors, course organisers, university staff, deanery staff, mentors, health librarians, trust staff, appraisers, College representatives) should be aware of good practice in the giving of careers information, advice and guidance and career counselling, and be able to signpost doctors to relevant sources of help.

The deanery needs to enable and ensure that all staff in educationally supportive posts are competent for their roles. There should be coaching skills and careers guidance skills development available for educational supervisors.

All those providing careers support should be well trained and supported themselves – with access to help and advice in their roles.

Taster career opportunities

The deanery should create opportunities for doctors to sample alternative careers or diversify within their chosen career. These might take the form of 'taster' rotations of various career specialties.

The deanery/trust should maintain an overview of doctors' career pathways

All trainees should keep the deanery or trust informed of their plans and progress to enable co-ordination of workforce planning, creation of careers opportunities etc.

Proactive retention

Trained doctors should be proactively retained by:

*   retraining
*   sabbaticals
*   educational and development programmes for those doctors who might otherwise leave the profession
*   proactive seeking of doctors not in NHS work.

Devise an implementation plan

As for any strategy, it is easier to draw up the strategy, than to make and implement the plan across the area to which it applies. Your initial flush of enthusiasm in drawing up the strategy will wane, and it will be difficult to sustain commitment without adequate resources, capacity and milestones that trigger successive deadlines.

So, to implement your strategy the following steps may be relevant:

*   consult widely in drawing up the strategy in the first place; draw in local champions and those who have responsibility for doctors' careers, recruitment and retention, performance, new roles etc
*   base your strategy on national recommendations[1]

- consult widely on drawing up your implementation plan using the networks established in evolving the strategy
- consider models of careers support in other professions that you can learn from e.g. legal profession
- cost the options in the draft implementation plan
- create options that give other bodies a part to play, to spread responsibility for implementing the plan as widely as possible, encourage others' contributions (e.g. provide job opportunities, bursaries, web resources) and sustain momentum
- seek resources for the preferred implementation plan: allocate funds from the deanery or trust budgets
- harness helpers and champions
- set up careers information online
- commission or provide training to educators or deanery/trust personnel to provide careers information or signpost doctors to it
- involve other 'stakeholders', e.g. medical schools to plan how the strategy will apply to them: recruiting school children and other graduates, for students *in situ* etc
- action your full project plan with detailed activities, expected outcomes, statement of assumptions and risks and how these will be predicted and addressed, milestones, resources etc.

Reference

1 Modernising Medical Careers Working Group for Career Management (2005) *Career Management: an approach for medical schools, deaneries, royal colleges and trusts*. The Stationery Office, London.

Appendix 1: Sources of information relating to careers and NHS matters, for all working with and for the NHS

- *British Council*, Bridgewater House, 58 Whitworth Street, Manchester M1 6BB. Information centre tel: +44 (0)161 957 7755. www.britishcouncil.org
  Offers personal advice on study options and opportunities in UK. Resources include information on courses, qualifications, institutions, English requirements, visas and travel. It has many offices in UK and worldwide.

- *Chartered Institute of Personnel and Development*, 151 The Broadway, London SW19 1JQ. Tel: +44 (0)20 8612 6200. www.cipd.co.uk
  Services provided include promotion of programmes, management consultation and training, guides on career management in organisations and counselling at work. It provides references for reports, articles and books about careers support.

- *Department of Health*. www.dh.gov.uk

- *Graduate Prospects*. www.prospects.ac.uk
  Graduate careers website, includes prospects planner which asks questions about skills, interests and motivations to generate job suggestions.

- *International Health Exchange/Red R*, 1 Great George Street, London SW1P 3AA. Tel : +44 (0)20 7233 1100. www.ihe.org.uk
  This is a charity assisting aid and development organisations to recruit qualified health professionals, through recruitment, training and works with agencies and individuals worldwide.

- *Learn Direct*, PO Box 900, Manchester M60 3LE. Tel: +44 (0)800 100 900. www.learndirect-advice.co.uk
  A national advice organisation offering general careers advice and information. You can call an advice line to discuss career options.

- *Médecins Sans Frontières (MSF)*. www.msf.org
  Medical volunteers recruitment for projects overseas.

- *Merlin*, 4th Floor, 56–64 Leonard Street, London EC2A 4LT. www.merlin.org.uk
  Recruits medical volunteers. Aims to provide immediate response to medical emergencies throughout the world.

- *NHS Alliance*, Goodbody's Mill, Albert Road, Retford, Nottinghamshire DN22 6JD. Tel: +44 (0)1777 869080. www.nhsalliance.org
  Representative organisation of primary care.

- *NHS Careers*, PO Box 376, Bristol BS99 3EY. Tel: +44 (0)845 6060655. www.nhscareers.nhs.uk
  Website gives information and national/local contact details.

- *National Primary and Care Trust Development Programme (NatPaCT).* www.natpact. nhs.uk
  Provided organisational development support to PCTs. NatPaCT programme closed 31 May 2005. Website no longer updated. Visit new sites at www. networks.nhs.uk and www.primarycarecontracting.nhs.uk

- *NHS Professionals.* Recruitment line: +44 (0)845 6060 345. www. nhsprofessionals.nhs.uk
  Aims to maximise the potential of doctors, nurses and corporate staff with support and flexibility to meet their own personal needs. Has guidance on flexible career schemes, training for lifelong learning etc.

- *Open University Careers Advisory Service.* www.open.ac.uk
  Practical resources to assist any student or graduate to make the right move: www.open.ac.uk/careers

- *Salomons Centre for Leadership and Management Development,* Broomhill Road, Southborough, Tunbridge Wells, Kent TN3 0TG. Tel: +44 (0)1892 507635. www.salomonsclmd.co.uk
  Able to provide psychometric and other instruments for self-awareness (Myers Briggs, MBTI, ABLE etc). Also specialise in the education, training and development of health professionals.

- *Society for Academic Primary Care (SAPC),* 4 Manor Farm Barns, Church Lane, Charlton-on-Otmoor, Oxon OX5 2UA. Tel: +44 (0)1865 331839. www.sapc. ac.uk
  Aims to promote excellence in research and education in general practice and primary healthcare.

- *Voluntary Services Overseas,* 317 Putney Bridge Road, London SW15 2PN. Tel: +44 (0)20 8780 7500. www.vso.org.uk
  Recruits volunteers for projects overseas, to share skills and learning and jointly achieve change.

- *Windmills Virtual Career Coach.* www.windmillsprogramme.com
  Provides virtual career coach, career fitness check and tactics for success.

Appendix 2: Sources of careers-related information for doctors

- *Academy of Medical Royal Colleges*, 1 Wimpole Street, London W1G 0AE. Tel: +44 (0)20 7408 2244. www.aomrc.org.uk
  Contains contact details and links to all Royal Colleges.

- *Association for the Study of Medical Education (ASME)*, 12 Queen Street, Edinburgh EH2 1JE. Tel: +44 (0)131 225 9111. www.asme.org.uk
  ASME is a membership organisation for doctors and educators from any clinical specialty and level. It offers careers guidance and personal development for healthcare professionals.

- *British International Doctors' Association*, 316A Buxton Road, Great Moor, Stockport SK2 7DD. Tel: +44 (0)161 456 7828.
  Provides counselling and careers advice for ethnic minority doctors and dentists. Works to protect and promote the interests of ethnic minority doctors and dentists working in the UK.

- *British Medical Association (BMA)*, BMA House, Tavistock Square, London WC1H 9JP. Tel: +44 (0)20 7387 4499. www.bma.org.uk
  The BMA represents doctors from all branches of medicine all over the UK, keeping members up to date with clinical and other medical issues. The science and education department provides information on the different agencies and advisers you may wish to contact in seeking solutions to career problems.

- *BMA Counselling*. Tel: +44 (0)8459 200169.
  24-hour counselling service for BMA members and their families. Confidential, professional help with work-related, emotional and personal problems.

- *BMA International Department*, BMA House, Tavistock Square, London WC1H 9JP. Tel: +44 (0)20 7383 6033/6793. www.bma.org.uk/international
  Advises overseas doctors on working in the UK and members on working abroad.

- *BMJ Careers Focus*, BMA House, Tavistock Square, London WC1H 9JR. Tel: +44 (0)20 7383 6125. www.bmjcareers.com
  Provides careers information and advice for medics with personal articles. Advertises jobs, courses; advice for overseas applicants and disabled doctors.

- *BMJ Chronic Illness Matching Scheme*. www.bmjcareers.com/chill
  Provides opportunity for doctors who have a chronic illness or disability to receive informal careers advice from another doctor.

- *BMJ Learning*. www.bmjlearning.com

- *Conference of Postgraduate Medical Deans*, 20 Guilford Street, London WC1N 1DZ. Tel: +44 (0)20 7692 3197. www.copmed.org.uk
  Gives contact details of all UK deaneries.

- *Doctors' Support Line*. Tel: +44 (0)870 765 0001. www.doctorssupportline.org
  Independent, confidential and anonymous helpline with all calls answered by volunteer doctors. Offers peer support. Available to all doctors to discuss

issues of work or personal concerns relating to their health, work or relation-ships.

- *Doctors' Support Network*, 38 Harwood Road, Fulham, London SW6 4PH. Tel: +44 (0)870 321 0642. www.dsn.org.uk
  Self-help group for doctors with mental health problems.

- *Faculty of Accident and Emergency Medicine*, 35–43 Lincoln's Inn Fields, London WC2A 3PE. Tel: +44 (0)20 7405 7071. www.emergencymed.org.uk/FAEM

- *Faculty of Dental Surgery*, Royal College of Surgeons, 35–43 Lincoln's Inn Fields, London WC2A 3PE. Tel: +44 (0)20 7405 3474. www.rcseng.ac.uk/dental/fds

- *Faculty of Occupational Medicine of the Royal College of Physicians*, 6 St Andrew's Place, Regent's Park, London NW1 4LB. Tel: +44 (0)20 7317 5890. www.facoccmed.ac.uk

- *Faculty of Public Health Medicine of the Royal College of Physicians*, 4 St Andrew's Place, London NW1 4LB. Tel: +44 (0)20 7935 0243. www.fphm.org.uk

- *General Medical Council (GMC)*, Regent's Place, 350 Euston Road, London NW1 3JN. Tel: +44 (0)845 357 8001. www.gmc-uk.org
  The GMC's aim is to maintain the standards of doctors that the public expect.

- *International Fellowship Scheme.* http://fellowships.tmpw.co.uk/index.asp

- *International Medical Recruitment.* www.internationalrecruitment.nhs.uk

- *Joint Committee on Postgraduate Training for General Practice (JCPTGP).* www.jcptgp.org.uk (ceased operating at September 2005).

- *Medical Forum*, 24 Woodlands, Overton, Hants RG25 3HN. Tel: +44 (0)705 007 7171. www.medicalforum.com
  Provides career guidance, professional growth and personal development for medical and dental professions. Offers personalised careers guidance and re-sources to learn how to compose a career plan.

- *Medical Practitioners' Union (MPU)*, 40 Bermondsey Street, London SE1 3UP. Tel: +44 (0)20 7939 7000. www.mpunion.org.uk
  MPU is a medical organisation that recognises the political issues of poverty, environments, living and working conditions, which need to be addressed if the health of the population is to be improved.

- *Medical Research Council*, 20 Park Crescent, London W1B 1AL. Tel: +44 (0)20 7636 5422. www.mrc.ac.uk
  The MRC's major forms of support are research grants and awards for training and research career development, covering all stages of a research career.

- *Medical Women's Federation*, Tavistock House North, Tavistock Square, London WC1H 9HX. Tel: +44 (0)20 7387 7765. www.medicalwomensfederation.org.uk
  Aims to advance the personal and professional development of women in medi-cine. Updates and informs members of changes affecting the medical profession and women's health issues. Offer members advice and support in their careers.

- *Modernising Medical Careers (MMC)*, 6th Floor, New Kings Beam House, 22 Upper Ground, London SE1 9BW. Fax: +44 (0)20 7633 7413. www.mmc.nhs.uk

MMC aims to improve patient care by delivering modernised and focused career structure for doctors through a major reform of postgraduate medical education. Also aims to provide careers advice and support for doctors at every stage of their career.

- *National Advice Centre for Postgraduate Medical Education*, PO Box 2516, St James House, Bristol BS2 2AA. Tel: +44 (0)117 915 7069. www.nhscareers.nhs.uk/nacpme
  Provides accurate and easily accessible information on topics relevant to overseas-qualified doctors intending to train and study in the UK.

- *National Association of Clinical Tutors (NACT)*, 56 Queen Anne Street, London W1G 8LA. Tel: +44 (0)20 7317 3109. www.nact.org.uk
  NACT aims to promote and develop postgraduate medical education. It represents and supports clinical tutors at national and regional level.

- *National Association of Sessional GPs (NASGP)*, PO Box 188, Chichester, West Sussex PO19 2ZA. Tel: +44 (0)1243 536428. www.nasgp.org.uk
  Offers general support to GP non-principals around their careers.

- *National Office for Summative Assessment*, 19 Buckingham Street, London WC2N 6EF. Tel: +44 (0)20 7484 2745. www.nosa.org.uk
  Website offers 24 hour a day information and downloads.

- *NHS Pensions Agency*. Helpline: +44 (0)1253 774440. www.nhspa.gov.uk

- *NHS Professionals*. Recruitment line: +44 (0)845 6060 345. www.nhsprofessionals.nhs.uk
  Aims to maximise the potential of all available doctors with the support and flexibility to meet their own personal needs. Gives guidance on flexible career schemes, training for lifelong learning, returner scheme etc.

- *Postgraduate Medical Education and Training Board*, Hercules House, Hercules Road, London SE1 7DU. Tel: +44 (0)20 160 6100. www.pmetb.org.uk

- *Rose*. www.rose.nhs.uk
  An NHS led site to support refugee and overseas qualified health professionals.

- *Royal College of Anaesthetists*, 48–49 Russell Square, London WC1B 4JY. Tel: +44 (0)20 7813 1900. www.rcoa.ac.uk

- *Royal College of General Practitioners (RCGP)*, 14 Princes Gate, Hyde Park, London SW7 1PU. Tel: +44 (0)20 7581 3232. www.rcgp.org.uk
  RCGP faculties might provide careers support.

- *Royal College of Obstetricians and Gynaecologists*, 27 Sussex Place, Regent's Park, London NW1 4RG. Tel: +44 (0)20 7772 6200. www.rcog.org.uk

- *Royal College of Ophthalmologists*, 17 Cornwall Terrace, London NW1 4QW. Tel: +44 (0)20 7935 0702. www.rcophth.ac.uk

- *Royal College of Paediatrics and Child Health*, 50 Hallam Street, London W1W 6DE. Tel: +44 (0)20 7307 5600. www.rcpch.ac.uk

- *Royal College of Pathologists*, 2 Carlton House Terrace, London SW1Y 5AF. Tel: +44 (0)20 7451 6700. www.rcpath.org

- *Royal College of Physicians*, 11 St Andrew's Place, Regent's Park, London NW1 4LE. Tel: +44 (0)20 7935 1174. www.rcplondon.ac.uk

- *Royal College of Physicians and Surgeons of Glasgow*, 232–242 St Vincent Street, Glasgow G2 5RJ. Tel: +44 (0)141 221 6072. www.rcpsglasg.ac.uk

- *Royal College of Physicians of Edinburgh*, 9 Queen Street, Edinburgh EH2 1JQ. Tel: +44 (0)131 225 7324. www.rcpe.ac.uk

- *Royal College of Psychiatrists*, 17 Belgrave Square, London SW1X 8PG. Tel: +44 (0)20 7235 2351. www.rcpsych.ac.uk

- *Royal College of Radiologists*, 38 Portland Place, London W1B 1JQ. Tel: +44 (0)20 7636 4432. www.rcr.ac.uk

- *Royal College of Surgeons of Edinburgh*, Nicolson Street, Edinburgh EH8 9DW. Tel: +44 (0)131 527 1600. www.rcsed.ac.uk

- *Royal College of Surgeons of England*, 35–43 Lincoln's Inn Fields, London WC2A 3PE. Tel: +44 (0)20 7405 3474. www.rcseng.ac.uk

- *Royal Institute of Public Health*, 28 Portland Place, London W1B 1DE. Tel: +44 (0)20 7580 2731. www.riph.org.uk

- *Royal Medical Benevolent Fund*. www.rmbf.org

- *Royal Pharmaceutical Society*, 1 Lambeth High Street, London SE1 7JN. Tel: +44 (0)20 7735 9141. www.rpsgb.org.uk

- *Royal Society of Medicine*, 1 Wimpole Street, London W1G 0AE. Tel: +44 (0)20 7290 2900. www.rsm.ac.uk

- *Royal Society of Tropical Medicine and Hygiene*, 50 Bedford Square, London WC1B 3DP. Tel: +44 (0)20 7580 2127. www.rstmh.org

- *Sick Doctors Trust*. Tel: +44 (0)870 444 5163. www.sick-doctors-trust.co.uk Helps and advises doctors who are suffering from the effects of addiction to alcohol and other drugs.

- *Support4Doctors*. www.support4doctors.org Aims to put doctors and their families in touch with organisations who can help.

- *UK Medical School Guide*. www.medschoolguide.co.uk

- *Women in Surgical Training (WIST)*, c/o Royal College of Surgeons, 35–43 Lincoln's Inn Fields, London WC2A 3PE. www.rcseng.ac.uk/career/wist/ WIST promotes surgery as a career for women and enables women who have chosen a career in surgery to realise their professional goals.

Armed forces

- *Defence Postgraduate Medical Deanery*, ICT Centre, Birmingham Research Park, Vincent Drive, Edgbaston, Birmingham B15 2SQ. Tel: +44 (0)121 415 8152.

- *Director Army General Practice*, Army Medical Directorate, The Former Army Staff College, Slim Road, Camberley, Surrey GU15 4NP. Tel: +44 (0)1276 412726.

- *Command Medical Officer (General Practice) (RAF)*, Room G67, Building 255, HQ PTC, RAF Innsworth, Gloucester GL3 1EZ. Tel: +44 (0)1452 712612 ext 6558.

- *Adviser GP Royal Navy*, PMO HMS Drake, Devonport, Plymouth PL2 2BG. Tel: +44 (0)1752 555401.

Appendix 3: Example of career development skills and techniques – one day workshop

Purpose

To give doctors with a management, educational or appraisal role the understanding and skills to promote career planning to Foundation Years doctors and medical colleagues, and to provide information and advice about career choices and development.

Outcomes of the workshop

- Understanding of the concepts and techniques of career planning.
- Recognition of when career planning will be effective for others.
- Understanding of the nature of careers information and guidance you can provide to other doctors.
- Introduction to the concepts and techniques of careers information and guidance.
- Realisation of the various competencies you need to provide careers information and guidance.
- Draft personal development plan to develop your competence as a provider of careers support and gather evidence of competence.

Programme

9.00 am: Coffee and networking
9.30 am: Introductions and welcome; purpose of the workshop
10.00 am: Overview of career planning from individual student's or doctor's perspective:

- context of NHS: *ad hoc* career planning, link between motivated/fulfilled workforce and performance
- job and career satisfaction
- where are you now?
- where do you want to be?
- how will you get there?
- what local/national services will help you make career choices?
- self-assessment of skills, aptitudes, values and career preferences and matching with own career
- understanding yourself, will enable you to help others more effectively

11.00 am: Coffee break
11.15 am: Considering your role in providing support for students or doctors in relation to their career choices, planning and development – as part of educational, appraisal or management remit:

- career management
- careers information
- careers advice/guidance
- career counselling.

Competencies: delivered as plenary with sharing of the descriptions of competence. In small groups, discuss how these relate to the individual, what gaps they might have, how they can gather evidence of competence. Then plenary.

12.15 pm:	Schein anchors. How these relate to you
1.00 pm:	Lunch
1.45 pm:	Active listening: a revision
2.05 pm:	Role-play – in trios – scenarios to reflect the providing of careers information, advice and guidance (each of trio plays observer, provider of careers support and GP receiving career support once) to:

- an appraisee who is confused as to whether to continue in practice
- a newly qualified doctor who is uncertain about their career specialty
- an established doctor who is asking for advice about diversifying their career.

Run as 15-minute role-play (realtime), followed by 10 minutes' discussion. After each role-play all complete an exercise assessing knowledge and skill needs of doctor participant playing provider of careers support.
    Reflect on use of careers support techniques and transferable skills:

- encouragement of career planning
- creation of rapport
- active listening
- good communication in general
- encouragement of others' self-analysis
- knowing where others should go for further information
- referring others to career counselling, coaching, a particular careers specialty

3.20 pm:	Coffee break
3.35 pm:	Discussion re learning points from role-play:

- did you provide careers information, advice/guidance, counselling?
- perceived knowledge and skill needs + whether or not verified by observer – agreement
- pool extent of knowledge/skills needs
- knowledge and skill gaps – capture in your personal development plan

4.00 pm:	Linking strategic approach in trust/deanery/SHA to vacancies, careers developments alongside planning service improvements: what you think the trust/deanery/SHA requires to do to support you? What careers information will you need to draw on?
4.30 pm:	Close

Index